ECTION

PREVENTION, HEALTH AND BRITISH POLITICS

To Rebecca, Emily and Hannah

30,- N/N

Prevention, Health and British Politics

Edited by

MIKE MILLS
Centre for the Study of Political Change
Department of Politics and Government
London Guildhall University

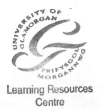

Learning Resources
Centre

Avebury

Aldershot · Brookfield USA · Hong Kong · Singapore · Sydney

Published by
Avebury
Ashgate Publishing Limited
Gower House
Croft Road
Aldershot
Hants GU11 3HR
England

Ashgate Publishing Company
Old Post Road
Brookfield
Vermont 05036
USA

British Library Cataloguing in Publication Data

Prevention, Health and British Politics
    I. Mills, Mike
    362.10941

ISBN 1 85628 190 6

Printed and Bound in Great Britain by
Athenaeum Press Ltd, Newcastle upon Tyne.

Contents

Acknowledgements

This book has been a long time in the making. It began as a germ of an idea in 1987-8 and has been nurtured by many people over the past five or six years. I would like to acknowledge the help given by the Nuffield Foundation which financed a conference of the authors at the City of London Polytechnic (as was) in September 1991. This contributed greatly to the final product and I am happy to advertise the Foundation's help. I would also like to thank Renee Gerson (my Head of Department) who has encouraged the project throughout and has placed the facilities of the Department at my disposal and given financial support to the author's conference.

The contributors have been good to work with and, putting aside the occasional panic over deadlines, I have enjoyed working with them. They, too, deserve my thanks for their patience and attention. I would particularly like to thank Michael Saward and Hugh Ward who made valuable comments on earlier drafts of the *Introduction* and Dermot McCann for his comments on the *Conclusion*. Elizabeth Bomberg and John Peterson have asked me to mention the help they received from Rod Rhodes in the writing of their chapter and I am pleased to do this.

I must also mention Chrissie, Colin, Daniel and Josh because I completely forgot them last time.

Lastly, I want to thank my family who ask very little of me and get less than they deserve in return. It is to my children (Rebecca, Emily and Hannah) that the book is dedicated.

Mike Mills

May, 1993

Contributors

Judith Allsop is Professor of Health Policy at South Bank University. She has written a number of books and articles on health policy including *Health Policy and the NHS*, *Changing Primary Care* and with Annabelle May, *the Emperor's New Clothes, FPC's in the 1980s*. She is a member of a health authority in London.

Elizabeth Bomberg is an EC specialist in the Department of Political Studies, University of Stirling, Scotland. She is author of *The Greening of the European Community* (Routledge, 1994) and numerous publications on EC environmental policies.

Richard Freeman graduated from the University of Oxford in 1986 with an honours degree in Modern History and Modern Languages. He took a Diploma in Social Policy at the University of Manchester, where he remained as a research student until 1991. He taught at both Machester Polytechnic and the University of Manchester, and is currently a lecturer in social policy in the Department of Political Science and Social Policy at the University of Dundee.

Alison Hann is a post-graduate student at the University of East Anglia with an interest in feminist theory and political science. The academic life suits her better than any of her previous occupations (including being a housewife and mother) because it's indoor work with no heavy lifting.

K.L. Lane has taught Australian and British politics, sociological theory and political philosophy at Flinders University, Australia, the Open University, Den Haag and Cambridge, and at Essex University. Her research interests include broadcasting and birthing. She is the mother of two children.

Mike Mills is Lecturer in Politics and Government at London Guildhall University. He is the author of *The Politics of Dietary Change* and his research interests include policy networks, environmental politics and public health. He is currently co-editing a book on neo-liberalism.

John Peterson lectures on the European Community in the Department of Politics, University of York. He is the author of *Europe and America in the 1990s: Prospects for Partnership* (Edward Elgar, 1993) and *High Technology and the Competition State: An Analysis of the Eureka Initiative* (Routledge, 1993).

Melvyn D. Read is a lecturer at The Queen's University of Belfast. His interests are with health, particularly the tobacco industry, and with the British Parliament. He has written on the tobacco industry and was a co-author of *Private Members Bills* with Professor David Marsh. He is currently involved in a project to build a data base on the voting behaviour of MPs on crucial votes in the House of Commons.

Michael Saward is Lecturer in Public Administration at Royal Holloway, University of London. He is author of *Co-optive Politics and State Legitimacy* and has published articles in various areas of democratic theory. His research interests are democratic theory, policy networks and green politics.

John Street is Lecturer in Politics and Director of the Centre for Public Choice Studies at the University of East Anglia. He is the author of *Rebel Rock: The Politics of Popular Music, Politics and Technology* and co-author of *Deciding Factors in British Politics*.

Hugh Ward is Senior Lecturer in Government at Essex University. His research interests include rational choice theory and environmental politics and he has published widely in these areas both in Britain and abroad.

1 Introduction

Mike Mills

It is, perhaps, a little unfashionable nowadays to isolate the preventive aspect of health care from the armoury of strategies that make up a more holistic, integrated approach. The new public health movement, for example, deliberately sets out to integrate policies which are curative, diagnostic and preventive. The essence of modern thinking on health care, which has been encapsulated in the World Health Organisation's *Global Strategy of Health For All by the Year 2000* (WHO, 1981) and the *Ottowa Charter for Health Promotion* (WHO, 1986), argues for a much greater plurality of methods to be used to manipulate services, behaviour and environments in order to augment health. This approach is free, by and large, of the more dogmatic attachments to single strategies which were more evident in the 1970s. At the root of this more holistic approach, however, is the assumption that each part of the restorative or preventive process is dependent upon the others, that to augment the general level of well being in the population, or to encourage the population to augment its own health, we cannot rely exclusively upon either doctors, nurses, hospitals or our own lifestyles. Rather, health strategies in the 21st century will not embody, as past strategies have, the belief that the environmental, social, economic or cultural causes of ill-health can be remedied within the institutional settings of hospitals or doctors surgeries.

A cursory glance at the most basic definitions of public health and health promotion will be enough to demonstrate the position of prevention in these strategies:

> (public health is ...) the science and art of preventing disease,
> prolonging life and promoting health through organised efforts
> of society (DHSS, 1988, p. 1).

Griffiths and Adams argue that health promotion:

> ... is generally agreed to take in three main kinds of activity
> ...: health education ...; prevention of ill-health - measures to
> reduce risk ...; legal fiscal and political measures, regulations,
> policies or voluntary codes to prevent ill-health and/or enhance
> well-being...(Griffiths and Adams, 1991, pp. 220-221).

There are two important points which need to be made here. The first is that prevention is clearly a central element of public health and health promotion, a point that hardly needs to be laboured. The second is that the range of policies which may be subsumed under these labels is very broad indeed because most aspects of public policy can, and do, have a health aspect to them. Importantly, however, it is the need to *prevent* ill-health which is responsible both for broadening the policy base of health care strategies and, conversely, shifting our focus away from orthodox health care systems. Prevention is the reason why health care cannot be confined to one isolated part of the political system. Not only are we justified, then, in examining prevention because it is part of a more systemic approach to health where strategies are interdependent, but it is clear that the need to prevent brings with it a great deal of political baggage which infringes upon policies areas where health may not be the first consideration.

This book begins with the assumption, therefore, that health strategies can no longer be confined to the systems of health care designed largely to cure or restore individuals. Consequently we cannot look only to the power of health professionals, their knowledge base, managerial systems etc. to evaluate or explain how we deal with health in a political context. The essence of prevention is that it is a pervasive concept which does not lend itself to single strategies or institutional settings. The diversity of the policy areas covered in this book is testimony to this.

But does this diversity preclude the possibility that we can generalise about the nature of prevention or preventive policies? Do concepts which are normally associated with prevention (risk and vulnerability for example) help us to explain across policy areas? What are the political constraints and opportunities which an essentially preventive health strategy faces? Do certain types of prevention have greater political mileage than others? To be able to answer questions like this we need to represent, as far as is possible, the types of issues that prevention addresses and then explore the factors which inform the political choices which are made. The collection of cases here attempts to do this.

Prevention - meaning and strategies

The prevention of disease or illness is not a new phenomena. Much of the public health revolution in the nineteenth century was preventive in character and many programmes aimed particularly at expectant and nursing mothers, infants and children have been established in one form or another for most of this century. The school meals service, school doctor and dentists services and health visiting, for example, all date from before the first world war. By and large, though, the current interest in prevention dates from the late 1960s and the 1970s and is marked by a particular interest in health problems which were thought at the time to be peculiarly 'modern', endemic and pervasive.

What distinguishes the emerging role of prevention in the 1970s is that it was seen as a more general strategy which was not confined to those groups which had historically been accepted as vulnerable. Its form and content were influenced by the types of health problems which the conventional system of institutionally-based health care had problems in resolving. It was clear, for example, that the most common causes of death (cancers, heart disease and accidents) were largely preventable but that orthodox medical intervention was unlikely ever to make significant inroads into the overall mortality figures (see, for example, Royal College, 1976). Similarly, it appeared as though many of these diseases could be attributed to personal lifestyle: we could give up smoking, drive more carefully, eat more sensibly, drink in moderation etc. It is not difficult to see why, when the Department of Health and Social Security (DHSS) tackled the subject of prevention (DHSS, 1977), the emphasis was upon what individuals could do for themselves. Despite the fact that this was also the time of the Primary Health Care Team, the community centre and the emergence of the community medicine as a model to compete (largely unsuccessfully) with bio-medicine, the emphasis remained upon lifestyle change. More recently, primary care has been reassessed (DHSS, 1987 and 1989; Allsop, 1989) and there has been a qualified shift away from a exclusive reliance upon individual lifestyle change (Williams, Calnan and Cant, 1991). A detailed account of these changes, and their prospects of success, is given by Allsop and Freeman in Chapter 2.

The character of prevention, then, is not defined only in terms of what people do for themselves, even though the politics of prevention in the 1980s might suggest this to be the case. As we saw above, there is more to prevention than lifestyle change and primary care and it is our job to disaggregate both the concept and the political context within which it now operates.

But the concept of prevention is a messy one. Most authors, including the then DHSS, believe there are three levels at which prevention can operate primary, secondary and tertiary - each of which correspond to the stages at which risks, or their effects, can be managed (DHSS, 1977). Primary prevention deals with things like immunisation, vaccination, health and safety at work, the control of pollution, diet, alcohol and smoking. The essence of this approach is that we can avoid or manipulate risks so that they do not adversely affect our health in the first place. Secondary prevention effectively concedes that avoiding or manipulating all risks is going to be impossible and so sees the early diagnosis of disease as a means of preventing a condition getting any worse and/or preventing its recurrence - this would normally include screening for example. Finally there is tertiary prevention which 'aims to reduce the burden of disability' (Ashton and Seymour,1988) and which would include all medical intervention given once a condition had been diagnosed.

This, of course, is an extremely broad definition of prevention which implies that all actions directed towards avoiding death, illness or injury are preventive in some sense or another. Commentators have pointed out that tertiary prevention, by any meaningful measure, is treatment, not prevention (Acheson, 1988). Without making the distinction between treatment and prevention it is, of course, very difficult to distinguish between prevention and cure.

It is perhaps inevitable that using the term prevention will lead us into problems of this sort. To prevent suggests a deliberate intervention in a causal process (Billis, 1981) which may begin with potential risks to the health of individuals, groups, communities, classes or populations (pollution, for example) and may end with death. In other words, we are all subject to risks of one sort or another which will do us harm if they are not controlled in some way. Definitionally, we have a problem because if we ask: 'at what point in this causal process do we try and control the risks or their consequences?' then any definition of prevention is going to struggle for a clear answer which can be universally applied. Is it always better, for example, to prevent the occurrence of risks or is it better to wait and deal with known symptoms? Can we say that the aim of prevention is to prevent death or morbidity, or is to prevent the occurrence and effects of risks much earlier in the causal process?

Logically we have to make the distinction between prevention and cure and this does not allow us to include tertiary prevention in any definition we use. Similarly, we cannot reasonably say that some points in the causal process are more preventive than others. We could maintain, for example, that it is more *sensible* to adopt a strategy which prevented or curtailed the availability or advertising of tobacco products rather than counselled people to give up, but we could not argue that one was prevention and one was not. What we could argue, under these circumstances, is that once the case for preventing smoking had been made we are entitled to say which type of preventive strategy is best, all things considered. Many of the case studies in this book work along these lines; they do not necessarily prescribe one type of prevention over and above another, but they often evaluate whether the strategy which is chosen will work.

On this basis it is reasonable to define preventive health policies as strategies designed to eliminate, detect, predict or manage societal risks which would otherwise have deleterious health consequences. Such a definition does distinguish between causes and effects, and prevention and cure, but does not and could not suggest the proper strategy of prevention.

This definition helps us to cut down on what we define as prevention to the extent that the treatment of conditions which already exist no longer qualify. But it retains, and emphasises, the pervasiveness of risks and the ways in which they may be managed. Consequently, many things which are done by governments, employers or individuals could be incorporated into a preventive health policy or might be seen as risk factors. Of course, some risks are seen as acceptable (driving a car, for example) and the costs of eliminating others might be prohibitive. We will not, of course, discover how these choices are made simply by defining prevention.

What we can do, though, is to notice that prevention (dealing with risks) is an open concept and leaves policy makers a great deal of political space. If we cannot pin prevention down in terms of the point at which governments should intervene, and we cannot prescribe any single strategy for prevention which is universally applicable, then we have to accept that we not only have many differing policy areas to contend with, but also, different ways in which health problems can be resolved.

It is particularly important for our purposes that we emphasise the degree of choice in preventive strategies because, by and large, these are political choices which reflect and promote aspects of our own political and economic values, our culture and our broader social system. It would be wrong, therefore, to believe that the most cost effective strategies are chosen on a largely impartial or objective basis. The evidence in the case studies here suggests that because prevention is such a pervasive issue which bumps up against so many highly charged political issues - ideology, patriarchy, economics, culture - the correlation between, for example, the level of risk and the commitment to prevention is actually very low. When we look more closely at what prevention entails it becomes a much more complicated, and certainly a less 'scientific', undertaking than we might expect.

It is generally thought that there are three distinct strategies for prevention - the individual, community and what we will call the systemic approach (Syme and Guralnik, 1988; Gray and Fowler, 1984). (1) It is here that we begin to get close to the more overtly political aspects of prevention and it is worth spending some time on each of these so that we can tease out the core political questions. These strategies are not mutually exclusive. Conceptually, it is usual to make the distinction but it is also usual to find that, in practice, the strategies reinforce one another and are often used together.

The individual approach

The individual approach focuses upon individual behaviour and individual lifestyles. Many societal risks, such as alcohol, food or cigarettes are activated through individual behaviour and it may not seem unreasonable, therefore, to see the individual as the site of preventive strategies. The assumption is that if behaviour is modified then many of the major causes of death or injury could be avoided altogether. Given that the three most common causes of death in Britain - heart disease, cancers and accidents - would all seem to benefit from this approach, and given also that in each of these cases conventional medicine cannot hope to deal with problems of this scale, then the individual approach would seem sensible. Of course, on the down-side, the individual approach is quite specific in where it allocates blame for its shortcomings. Ryan (1971) argued convincingly that the tendency within this approach is to 'blame the victim' if they fail to take the advice or information on offer, even though it may be difficult for them to do so. In other words, it assumes that the only responsibility for health stands with the individual even though they may be victims of the actions or inactions, policies or non-policies of others. Allsop and Freeman (chap.2), Read (chapter. 6) and Street (chap. 5) each demonstrate that this approach has a number of serious shortfalls and it is generally accepted that unless it is used in conjunction with a more supportive strategy, its use is more political than anything else. There is a great deal that can, and has, been said about the validity of the assumptions which govern this approach. We will return to these later.

Generally speaking this approach can work in one of two ways; either through health promotion/education campaigns which actively seek to change peoples behaviour, like those for heart disease, AIDS, smoking or heroin; or through the provision of information to the general public about the products they purchase, such as nutritional labels on food. In both cases the objective is broadly the same although the political mechanisms involved are quite different. Health education on a national scale is normally the preserve of the Health Education Authority (HEA) (formerly the

Health Education Council (HEC)) and at local or community level is done through health authorities and local authorities. Providing consumers with information about their purchases is either at the discretion of producers themselves or is dealt with by government and producers often on the advice of 'experts' coopted by government departments.

Increasingly, then, as we begin to disaggregate what an individual preventive strategy entails, it becomes clear that we are treading upon some sensitive political toes. As Mills and Saward will demonstrate in chapter 10, the individual approach fits neatly with liberal democratic notions of personal responsibility and a more minimalist role for the state. The state is only giving individuals information and perhaps a little encouragement and support, it is then up to them whether they wish to act on that advice. Indeed, the greater part of Britain's preventive policies in the latter half of the 1970s and early 1980s was predicated upon this advisory role for government (see following chapter for more detail). In large part governments took such an approach because it was felt that the state could not legitimately extend its responsibilities and interfere with, for example, personal consumption nor should it manipulate the supply of goods or simply because it was cheap. It is difficult to read *Prevention and Health* (DHSS, 1977) and the subsequent booklets in the Prevention and Health series, without concluding that successive governments have been acutely aware of what they perceive to be the legitimate boundaries of state action. Brand (1969) gives a very good example of how these types of arguments apply to the fluoridation of the water supply.

Of course, the ideological dimension can also work against the use of this particular strategy. Health education can be seen as social engineering and there can, and has, been immense pressure put on health education agencies to tone down their messages if they appear too prescriptive or promote health at the expense of other considerations such as those of producers (see, Farrent and Russell, 1985; Mills, 1992). Despite this, politically the individual approach is very popular and it is not difficult to see why. Not only does it tend to support an ideological view of the role of the state which is central to the British political system, but it is relatively inexpensive (the budget of the HEA is around about £30m per annum) and it has a high political profile. In later chapters, it will become clear that political profile and ideology are very important considerations in a number of different policy areas (Ward, chapter 8 (water purity), Street, chapter 5 (AIDS), Hann, chapter 3 (breast cancer screening), for example).

So, the evidence suggests that consumers of health education and goods offered for sale (just about everybody) are often caught up in a classic liberal dilemma, whereby the state is assumed to support the right of citizens to be informed on the one hand, and the right of producers to be free of punitive regulation, on the other.

The political nature of the individual approach is, therefore, quite clear. Any information given to the general public with the authority of a government agency is a political commodity. It can adversely affect the interests of some groups, can promote value conflicts and define what a legitimate role for the state and the individual might be as far as preventive health policies are concerned. We will see in later chapters (notably Street's chapter on AIDS) that it would be unwise to believe that the preventive message is unimpaired by political considerations or to believe that these considerations do not have a material effect on the messages themselves.

The community approach

One of the key aspects of health promotion, and a central tenet of public health in general, is the use of community-based preventive strategies. To take a community approach is not to ignore the individual or systemic aspects of prevention, but rather to support that action with services targeted on communities and to make full use of the plurality of agencies available to improve lifestyles, environments and services. The basic unit of analysis, therefore, is less the individual and more the communities, or groups within communities which are targeted. Many of these services are provided by the NHS in the form of general practice, mid-wifery, community nursing, ante and post natal services, health visiting, screening and so on. Local authority's Social Services Departments (SSD's) and Education Departments, for example, also contribute in terms of social work, school meals, occupational therapy, care of the elderly, and to a limited extent, school curicula. Similarly, councils at the district level are responsible for environmental health and housing.

There are good reasons to take such an approach to prevention. The evidence suggests (McCron and Budd, 1987, pp. 205-7) that while public information campaigns or health education are useful, their degree of success depends to a great extent on the quality of the community services available to support them. Equally, the community approach implies health strategies which are more tailored to the needs of particular communities. It may be true that all communities will need certain services (general practice, ante and post-natal services, for example) but communities with high levels of unemployment, a large ethnic minority community, or endemic drug-related problems, may need special support. In these cases, and many others, community based work has demonstrable preventive potential but relies to a great extent upon the knowledge base we have of the communities, the coordination of policies and services between and within agencies as well, of course, as resources.

Politically, we now have a different set of variables with which we must characterise prevention and which are more thoroughly covered by Allsop and Freeman below. The community approach is one which is largely *professionally administered* and so the politics of prevention will be affected by professional ideologies and territoriality. Indeed, it has been argued that the failure of primary care to blossom in the 1970s was the result of it failing to compete successfully with curative medicine once local authority responsibilities for prevention were transferred to the NHS in 1974 (Lewis, 1986). In chapter 4 Lane gives a very good example of how childbirth based upon a bio-medical model of health can not only compete with community-based strategies but effectively de-skill a profession (mid-wives) and institutionalise childbirth within hospitals. While this may be an extreme example, current reforms of both the NHS and the introduction of community care suggest similar competition particularly within the nursing profession. Equally, however, the community approach is characterised by *institutional and organisational cleavages*. The most obvious of these is between the NHS and local government, although the experiences of, for example, Oxford (Allen, 1992) and Liverpool (Ashton and Seymour, 1988) suggest that intra-agency factors are also very important. But the precise form of these institutions can also be a product of professional behaviour and there is certainly a reciprocal influence between professionals and the institutions within which they work. SSDs, for example, were the product of the successful professionalisation of social work (Webb and Wistow, 1987). Similarly, administrative and bureaucratic arrangements can also affect the power relations within them, as was the case of Community Physicians within the NHS (Lewis, 1986). In other words, we should not take institutions and the professions within them as neutral factors in the development or implementation of policies for each, to some extent, is the product of the other.

Now, the politics of the community approach is determined in large part by aspects of professionalisation and by the institutional fragmentation which has accompanied it but if we return to the idea that prevention is concerned with societal risks then it is clear that national and international level policy making has a crucial effect as well. In areas such as education, housing, social security and centre-local relations, the context of the community approach can be radically affected by decisions which are taken without the preventive aspects of social policies being borne in mind. For example, housing policy and the changes to housing benefits can affect employment prospects, homelessness, poverty, stress, respiratory problems, mobility and other factors correlated to health. It is no wonder, then, that publications associated with the new public health emphasise the interdependence of preventive strategies and see that the risks which the community approach seek to manage can seldom be eliminated by that approach alone. Of course, this is as true, if not more so, of the individual approach.

The systemic approach

The systemic approach, on the other hand, looks to manipulate the risks to which we are exposed by creating safer systems (or environments) for us to experience. We could include housing, the food supply, pollution and road safety in this category. These systems are inherently risky places and there are few actions we can take, or experiences we can have, which do not entail some level of risk. Some of these risks we can avoid ourselves, others we can be counselled over, but there are a range of cases which are beyond the scope of individual behaviour or professional intervention. We cannot affect the purity of our own water supply through changes in consumption, we are not in a position to regulate exhaust emissions, or to know if certain food additives are carcinogenic. In short the systemic approach assumes 1) that we are affected by systemic risks and 2) that these risks have to be eliminated, detected, predicted or managed on our behalf.

Broadly speaking the systemic approach incorporates three different roles for the state: the provision of public goods, for example, safe roads; the regulation of goods offered for consumption, for example, controls on the toxicity of food or the inclusion of seat belts in cars; and finally controlling the effects of production, that is, pollution or other externalities.

With the rise of the environmental movement in the late 1970s these systemic risks have been given greater political prominence not only because many are harmful to humans, but because they affect other species and sensitive ecological systems. As we would expect, given the range of policies the systemic approach incorporates, the types of health problem are also very varied, and the types of political mechanisms necessary to deal with them equally so. Doll and Peto (1981) have argued that perhaps as much as 80 per cent of cancers are preventable and many of these are likely to have a systemic origin. Similarly, heart disease, the major cause of mortality in many industrialised countries, appears to be a disease well grounded in patterns of consumption, lifestyle and stress all of which have a systemic aspect (DHSS, 1984). Other examples, such as those of asbestos or lead in petrol show that systems can have adverse health consequences.

Historically, policies related to product regulation and the regulation of the effects of production have been extremely fragmented. Much of this regulation is done between producers and departments of state and often has a strong technocratic component to it. The typical model of producer regulation sees government-industry relations as fairly secretive with very little accountability and public scrutiny. It also sees policy in general made in discrete sub-sectors with very little reference to other sub-sectors so the interests involved in policy making are well entrenched and there is little opportunity for other interests to have an input into policy. By and large, the Department of Health (DoH) is responsible for advising other departments on the health consequences of their policies although it is invariabley the case that where problems recur regularly, then the 'home' department will have their own advisers. Although DoH representatives are invited to attend the meetings of other departments as a matter of courtesy, their status in normally that of an observer. Read (chapter 6) gives us a good example of how this system works with the regulation of the tobacco industry. Similarly, industry is normally extremely well informed by its own experts. Consequently, there are often many sources and interpretations of scientific and medical evidence, each of which compete for the attention of policy makers - the paradigm case being the discrepancies, fostered by the food industry, of the evidence linking diet to health. Equally, even if we accept that the DoH has a meaningful advisory role on, say, the control of chemical carcinogens, we also have to accept that it will not be the DoH which eventually formulates and implements policy - that will be done elsewhere. In short, the greater the political fragmentation of decision making institutions, the greater the likelihood that prevention will simply be absorbed within the dominant policy style (and content) of the department which ultimately delivers policy. Bomberg and Peterson (chapter 9) provide a very similar type of argument when discussing prevention and the European Commission.

Inevitably, then, we cannot expect to see a linear progression from the advice of experts or technocrats through to public policy any more than we should expect our knowledge of risks to be an uncontentious political issue. It is often the case that advice is mediated through political, economic or ideological considerations. Even attempts by the British government to prevent heart disease have had to take into consideration the affects that large scale changes in saturated fat consumption would have on farmers, food manufacturers and food retailers (Mills, 1992). Ward (chapter 8) provides a convincing argument that the public investments in cleaning up the water supply were influenced as much by the imminent privatisation of the industry as they were by any adverse health consequences attributable to water. Read's chapter on smoking is an even more stark example of the political distance that can exist between societal risks and the public policies which address them. This is not to say that prevention is necessarily a good thing regardless of the costs involved, but it does indicate that there are strong politico-economic implications for the systemic regulation of the goods offered for sale.

The regulation of externalities gives us much the same sort of message as far as prevention is concerned. During the 1980s there has been a conscious attempt by successive governments to rationalise a system of regulation (which had evolved in a notoriously ad hoc way) through the creation of Her Majesties Inspectorate of Pollution (HMIP), the National Rivers Authority (NRA) and the Environmental Protection Act (Weale, O'Riordan and Kramme, 1991). Respectively these have attempted to integrate the agencies responsible for the regulation of stationary pollution and the control of the water supply and to strengthen the regulatory role of local authorities. Again, government-industry relations are an important political factor because the regulation of externalities is a process which is necessary primarily because of the actions of industry. Equally, the division of responsibilities between centre and periphery is also important. Allen (1991) argues that:

> Central Inspectorates have a role to play, but too often they are
> thin on the ground, lack local accountability and are not around
> when the problem occurs (Allen, 1991, 137).

Historically, the relationship between inspectorates and those they regulate has been a very comfortable one and has reflected the British approach to regulation more generally which has been flexible, informal and cooperative (Vogel, 1986). Inspectorates have been very reluctant to take polluters to court and have cherished the trusting and consensual nature of their policy implementation which did not apply universal regulatory standards. With the EC taking a greater part in regulation this is likely to change as universal standards are applied and the system has less flexibility although the Environmental Health Officers (EHO's) of local authorities have always tended to take a more adversarial approach to those they regulate.

   The politicisation of the environment and Britain's entry into the EC has meant that the systemic aspects of prevention have often had a high political profile and that the political agenda may be beyond of the control of the British government itself. However, the political considerations involved in policy making are pretty clear. *Producer interests*, within the broader regulatory network, are central actors and are valued by the state. This value rests not only on their ability to create wealth and employment, but also on the fact that there is some ideological compatibility between the liberal democratic values of the state and the market orientation of producers (see Mills and Saward, chapter 10). Many systemic health problems are related to key policy areas for any government - energy, agriculture and transport for example - and this simply adds to the *fragmentation* which is characteristic of this approach to prevention because policy not only fragments along institutional lines but also implies that many preventive health policies are in *competition* with other priority areas of public policy.

*   *   *   *   *

These, then, are the strategies of prevention and, interestingly, none of them support the idea that tertiary prevention - which by definition should work within the institutions of the health care system - is actually prevention. When we disaggregate the three approaches to prevention none give any indication that treatment falls within their strategies.

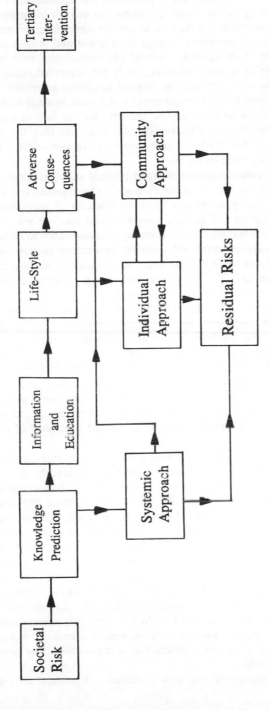

PRIMARY APPROACH

SECONDARY APPROACH

Societal Risk → Knowledge Prediction → Information and Education → Life-Style → Adverse Consequences → Tertiary Intervention

Systemic Approach

Individual Approach

Community Approach

Residual Risks

Primary Approach

Producer Interests
Dominant Ideology
Institutional Territoriality
Policy/Institutional
Fragmentation

Secondary Approach

Producer Interests
Dominant Ideology
Institutional Territoriality
Fragmentation
Constraints on Agency

Tertiary Intervention

Bio-Medical Model of Health
Professional Policy Control
Institutional fragmentation
Professional Cleavages

Diagrammatically the sites and strategies of prevention are represented in Figure 1. The diagram is as interesting for the things it does not tell us as it is for the things it does. Working on the assumption that the need to prevent comes from the existence of societal risks, the most basic preventive strategy is to detect and predict those risks before manipulating them at the systemic level. If this works, then risks have been successfully managed and if it does not work, or is not attempted, then we must assume either that we live with them because they are politically acceptable (more on this below) or that they have adverse consequences which must be dealt with by other preventive strategies. If, for whatever reason, the risks are not seen as systemically manipulable, as would be the case with smoking for example, then the individual approach would be tried, and such adverse consequences as remain would then be the responsibility of community based strategies.

At each point in the preventive process different political variables come into play, and these are indicated at the bottom of the diagram. The systemic and individual approaches are far more likely to infringe upon the interests of producers and the dominant ideological preferences of decision makers because they are not confined to the health care system alone but intrude into everyday politico-economic relationships. Similarly, their messages are pervasive and ideologically sensitive because they touch upon two central questions as far as the role of the state is concerned; how far should the state act on behalf of individuals and how does the state make the trade offs necessary between public health and private consumption?

The community approach, on the other hand, has historically been far more affected by; professional considerations; the predominance of the bio-medical model of health, which sees the individual as a largely passive recipient of medical intervention; and by the institutionalisation of the power of health, or other, professionals. The success of the bio-medical approach can in large part be attributed to the fact that it operates within a largely enclosed institutional framework and does not infringe upon broader structural interests in the way that much prevention does. Indeed, whichever approach to prevention is considered, it is interesting that the simple construction and separation of institutions can have a profound effect on the nature and likelihood of preventive health policies.

There are important points which are not represented in the diagram, and these will become evident in the case studies. Lane's chapter on childbirth, for example, demonstrates how the existence and nature of risks can be manipulated by those with a vested interest in portraying home-births as 'riskier' than hospital deliveries, even though the evidence suggests otherwise. How we perceive risks, and how we choose between them is not, therefore, a simple matter of objective assessment (Boehmer-Christiansen, 1988; Levine and Lilienfeld, 1987; Peters and Barker, 1993). In short, the very act of believing that a risk exists and attempting to gain knowledge of it is one which tells us as much about ourselves as it does about the thing we fear. Similarly, Ward argues that our perceptions of the risks posed by our water supply cannot be properly understood unless we take into consideration the cultural norms which affect our perceptions. Much the same story can be told for breast cancer screening (Hann, Chapter 3). The fear in which cancer is held in western countries, while clearly related to the risks of having it, is also a cultural fear of the unknown and untaken risk (Douglas and Wildavsky, 1982).

If the choice between preventive strategies is ultimately a political one, as is the choice of whether to prevent or not, then it is important to understand that we may wish to prevent those things we fear rather than those which do us the most harm, and we may embark on strategies which are neither cost-effective or necessary as a consequence.

Equally, even if we can agree that a particular health problem is worth preventing, our knowledge of the risk factors and our ability to detect and predict them is seldom as complete as we might like. Epidemiology, for example, is a notoriously costly and time consuming science which seldom produces results which are as unequivocal as policy makers would prefer (Levine and Lilienfeld, 1987). This type of problem is exacerbated when the evidence falls short of proof although, interestingly, less information does not necessarily mean less likelihood of prevention. Hann (chapter 3) and Ward (chapter 8) both argue that the evidence upon which policies for (respectively) breast cancer screening and water purification were based, was in fact quite weak but policies went ahead anyway. Of course, in the case of smoking the evidence is unequivocal and yet very little is done. It is these types of inconsistencies which will be addressed in the *Conclusion* to the book.

In short, prevention is a political commodity which can demonstrate many of the essential features both of liberal democracies in general and the British political system in particular. Health strategies which incorporate prevention, in part or in whole, will be crucially affected by variables and policy areas not normally associated with health but which will show how 'health' cannot be meaningfully pursued in institutional settings separated from the societal causes of risk.

The case studies

No single volume can do justice to the range of policy issues which can justifiably be labelled preventive health policies. The collection of essays here does, however, represent all the major themes which I have argued are important in any consideration of the politics of prevention.

Allsop and Freeman take us through the policies for prevention which have been in evidence in Britain over the past two decades and emphasise that, in comparison to other countries, Britain has been slow to respond to the WHO's programme *Health For All by the Year 2000*. They note the institutional and professional cleavages which exist in Britain for the formulation and delivery of preventive policies and give examples (alcohol, tobacco and health education) of preventive policies at work. They end by giving an assessment of recent reforms of the NHS in terms of their effects on prevention.

Hann describes for us the political and professional developments surrounding the introduction of mass mammography. Screening is a core aspect of secondary prevention, yet Hann argues that the evidence supporting the utility of mass mammography is far from convincing. Rather, she argues that it is far easier to explain its introduction in terms of the political context in which the decision was made, that is, 1) very close to the general election of 1987 and 2) with growing public concern over government inaction. Hann's case, therefore, provides a good example of how the pressure to 'do something' is a very real one.

Lane's chapter on childbirth gives a very good illustration of how the power relations within the NHS have had a notable impact upon the nature of community-based services (mid-wifery). Lane argues that the institutional arrangements of the NHS and the power base which this has afforded practitioners of the bio-medical model have defined preventive strategies in childbirth. These strategies reflect patriarchal and professional dominance and have succeeded in institutionalising childbirth when the health case for doing so remains to be made.

We then have two chapters that address issues which have strong elements of the individual approach. *Street's* chapter on AIDS sensitises us to how the timing and nature of policy can be affected by factors which are largely extraneous to the health problem itself. Street argues that the decision to launch the first phase of the AIDS education campaign was taken only when AIDS was seen as a threat to the heterosexual population and the preventive message that was eventually given was as much as a moral one as it can an educative one. He also argues that policies on AIDS competed with, and were affected by, values which were dominant in other policy areas (notably those on drug abuse) and that those policies were effectively captured by those with clinical skills.

The first of *Read's* two chapters considers smoking, which has been the object of all three preventive strategies. Read makes clear that it is very difficult to establish that Britain actually has an anti-smoking policy in any meaningful sense. He looks to the network of tobacco-based interests around the DoH as an indication of the success of the producers in constraining the actions of successive governments and he demonstrates the ways in which industry can attempt to influence both government and the political agenda. He demonstrates quite clearly that even though the success of the tobacco has been seen in 1) its power to mobilise Parliament in its defense and 2) its tax-raising role, the tobacco industry has many natural allies both in Parliament and the government.

Read's second chapter, on seat belts, is perhaps the best example in this book of how ideological factors, and in particular the freedom of the individual, can affect preventive strategies. He takes us through the discussions in Parliament which surrounded attempts to introduce the compulsory wearing of seat belts during the 1970s and the 1980s. We find that concern for individual freedom was a crucial feature of the debates and was largely responsible for the delay in introducing the legislation. We also find with seat belts, as we do with other preventive health policies, that these ideological objections have been put to one side once the benefits of constraining freedom appear to outweigh the costs.

The systemic approach to prevention is dealt with directly by *Ward* in his chapter on water purity. He argues that the issue of water safety has been influenced by the actions of environmental groups which have exploited both our cultural fear of impure water and the privatisation plans of the Conservative government. Ward suggests that even though the adverse health consequences associated with the water supply are, in comparative terms, not great it may still be rational to incur the expense of cleaning it up if we value its purity and if we wish to avoid adverse consequences in the future.

Bomberg and Peterson take us through the preventive role of the EC. Increasingly, the EC plays an important role in regulating the products offered for sale in Britain, the quality of the environment, research and development and will perhaps in the future regulate our social policies more directly as well. They argue that preventive policy making in the EC is fragmented and subject to the territoriality normally associated with bureaucratic organisations. However, they also argue that the Commission is not as susceptible to electoral short-termism as national governments and this makes for interesting comparisons between national and supra-national preventive policy making.

Mills and Saward's chapter on ideology introduces us to the ideological pathways which preventive policies have to tread. Liberal democracy, it is argued, values individualism, preserves market relationships and promotes patriarchal relationships. Consequently, the values represented in our political system tend to make some strategies easier than others, some groups more worthy of protection than others, as well as playing a leading role in defining what is or is not politically acceptable as far as prevention is concerned. The regularity with which the ideological aspects of liberal democracy affect the nature of preventive policies suggests that some discussion of it is central to any understanding of the political context within which preventive policies are made.

Conclusion

These cases are each interesting in themselves, but collectively they provide the opportunity for comparison and to search for common ground in the politics of prevention - this task is addressed in the *Conclusion* although there are preliminary observations which can be made here.

To be able to generalise across cases as diverse as these it is most likely that only macro-level variables such as ideology, economics, culture and institutions will hold in all or most cases. Of course, explaining only at the macro level, while necessary, will not give us everything we need. We need to incorporate meso-level concepts such as producer interests and professionals, and Street's chapter on AIDS suggests that the micro-level aspects of individual behaviour can also be important. Similarly, we need to test whether the concept of risk is actually very good at explaining or predicting prevention in a comparative context. And we need to be aware of the long journey that has to be taken from the perception of societal risk to the implementation of policies geared to eliminating, avoiding or managing those risks.

This book takes as its starting point the fact that a central feature of health care into the next century will be preventive in orientation. I have argued here that the strategies available to promote prevention each have political aspects to them which can affect their likely adoption or success. The politics of prevention implies competing professional orthodoxies; institutional cleavages; value judgements concerning the role of the state, the preservation of market sovereignty and the rationality and capability of the individual; judgements on who deserves support from the state; the political mediation of knowledge and much more besides.

To comment on prevention is, therefore, to comment not only on how we organise our health care services, but also on the values and institutions which govern us. The cases which follow are as diverse as the political system itself and suggest that the elimination, detection, prediction and management of societal risk cannot be understood without taking its political context into consideration.

Footnotes

1) We have chosen to use the term 'systemic' as opposed to 'environmental' approach to prevention because later chapters refer to environmental policy and we want to avoid confusion between the two.

Bibliography/references

Acheson, R.M. (1988), 'Prevention versus Cure:Use of Resources in the National Health Service', in, Keynes, M., Coleman, D.A. and Dimsdale, N.H., *The Political Economy of Health and Welfare*, Macmillan in association with the Eugenics Society, London.

Allen, P. (1991), 'Environmental Health Officers', in, Draper, P. (ed), *Health Through Public Policy: The Greening of Public Health*, Green Print, London.

Allen, P. (1992), *Off the Rocking Horse*, Green Print, London.

Allsop, J. (1989), 'Health', in, M. McCarthy (ed), *The New Politics of Welfare*, Macmillan, London.

Ashton, J. and Seymour, H. (1988), *The New Public Health*, Open University Press, Milton Keynes.

Billis, D. (1981), 'At Risk of Prevention', *Journal of Social Policy*, vol. 15, no.4, pp. 467-88.

Boehmer-Christiansen, S. (1988), 'Black Mist and Acid - science as a fig leaf of policy',*Political Quarterly*, vol. 59, pp. 145-60.

Brand, J.A. (1969), 'The Politics of Fluoridation: A Community Conflict', *Political Studies*, vol. XIX, no. 4, pp. 430-9.

DHSS (1977), *Prevention and Health*, Cmd 7047, HMSO, London.

DHSS (1984), *Diet and Cardiovascular Disease*, Report of the Committee on the Medical Aspects of Food Policy, HMSO, London.

DHSS (1987), *Promoting Better Health: The Government's Programme for Improving Primary Health Care*, Cmd 249, HMSO, London.

DHSS (1988), *Public Health in England: The Report of the Committee of Inquiry into the Future Development of the Public Health Function*, Cmd 289, HMSO, London.

DHSS (1989), *Working for Patients*, Cmd 555, HMSO, London.

Douglas, M. and Wildavsky, A. (1982), *Risk and Culture*, University of California Press, Berkeley.

Doll, R. and Peto, R. (1981), *The Causes of Cancer*, Oxford University Press, Oxford.

Farrent, W. and Russell, J. (1985), *The Politics of Health Information*, Bedford Way Papers 28, Institute of Education, University of London.

Gray, J.A. and Fowler, G. (1984), *Essentials of Preventive Medicine*, Blackwell Scientific Publications, London.

Levine, S. and Lilienfeld, A. (eds) (1987), *Epidemiology and Health Policy*, Tavistock Publications, London.

Lewis, J. (1986), *What Price Community Medicine*, Wheatsheaf Books, Brighton.

McCron, R. and Budd, J. (1987), 'Mass Communications and Health Education', in, Sutherland, I. (ed), *Health Education: Perspectives and Choices*, National Extension College, Cambridge.

Mills, M.P. (1992), *The Politics of Dietary Change*, Dartmouth, Aldershot.

Peters, G.G. and Barker, A. (1993), *Scientific Advice to Governments*, Edinburgh University Press, Edinburgh.

Royal College of Physicians of London and the Cardiac Society (1976), 'The Prevention of Coronary Heart Disease', *Journal of the Royal College of Physicians*, vol. 10, no.3, April.

Ryan, W. (1971), *Blaming the Victim*, Vintage Books, New York.

Syme, S.L. and Guralnik, J.M. (1987), 'Epidemiology and Health Policy:coronary heart disease', in, Levine, S. and Lilienfeld, A. (eds), *Epidemiology and Health Policy*, Tavistock Publications, London.

Vogel, D. (1986), *National Styles of Regulation*, Cornell University Press, Ithaca.

Weale, A., O'Riordan, T. and Kramme, L. (1991), *Controlling Pollution in the Round*, Anglo-German Foundation, London.

Webb, A and Wistow, G. (1987), *Social Work, Social Care and Social Planning*, Longman, London.

Williams, S., Calnan, M. and Cant, S. (1991), 'Health Promotion and Disease Prevention in the 1990s', *Medical Sociology News*, vol. 16, no. 3.

World Health Organisation (1981), *Global Strategy for Health For All by the Year 2000*, WHO, Copenhagen.

World Health Organisation, Health and Welfare Canada, Canadian Public Health Association (1986), *Ottowa Charter for Health Promotion*, WHO, Copenhagen.

2 Prevention in health policy in the United Kingdom and the NHS

Judith Allsop and Richard Freeman

This chapter gives an account of policies for the prevention of ill-health in the UK over the past two decades. Such policies have been slow to develop despite the poor health status of the population compared to other developed countries (OHE, 1992, Table 1.10, p. 25). Britain has lagged behind countries such as Sweden, Norway, the USA, Canada and New Zealand in adopting a strategic approach to prevention and in taking up the challenges of the World Health Organization's *Health For All by the Year 2000* programme. The chapter looks chronologically at national policies for prevention over the period 1970-90. A final section identifies the ideological, structural and political factors which may dilute the impact of the policies put forward in the government's recent discussion of *The Health of the Nation* (DoH, 1991, 1992). Two questions are addressed: what are the weaknesses of UK health policy in respect of prevention, and are the 1990 *Working for Patients* reforms and the proposals put forward in *The Health of the Nation* likely to bring any change in direction?

The place of prevention in the NHS

Although the preamble to the 1946 NHS Act which established the NHS gave equal weight to curing the sick, caring for the frail and disabled and preventing ill-health, there was little policy emphasis on the latter until the mid-1970s. Indeed, the first major reorganisation of the service in 1974 was concerned primarily with the integration of acute and community services and in fact diminished and fragmented the role of public health.

In the tripartite health service which existed from 1948 until 1974, public health had been part of the administrative responsibility of local authorities, and had been discharged through the Medical Officer of Health (MoH). These public health doctors were primarily concerned with the coordination and delivery of community health services. The focus of public health policy had shifted away from the classic problems of the urban environment in the early decades of the twentieth century. By the end of the 1960s the MoH seemed lost in time:

> Just as the public health doctor was not able successfully to justify his continued work in personal prevention, so he also failed to make a good case for the medical administration of welfare work. Thus MOsH increasingly found themselves accused of failure in respect to the delivery of effective community care and squeezed between the twin pressures of general practice from without and social work from within (Lewis, 1986, p. 59).

In consequence, a new occupational specialism of community medicine was created in 1974, effectively by no more than administrative fiat. This was part of the general 'organizational fix' (Klein, 1989) in welfare that included reform of the personal social services. The community physician held the parallel functions of giving specialist advice on public health both within the health district and to the local authority and of taking a lead in integrating the management of clinical medical services. The government viewed the community physician as a lynch-pin of the newly integrated NHS structure:

> There seems no doubt but that in the policy documents of 1972 the role of the community physician was envisaged primarily as a means of integrating the NHS and of achieving effective consensus management (Lewis, 1986, p. 117).

On the local authority side, however, reorganisation served to downgrade prevention and rob it of medical leadership just as it was beginning to rise up the policy agenda. Within health districts it placed the community physician (acting as District Medical Officer) in a difficult role. The specialism of community medicine ranked low in the medical hierarchy and community physicians lacked both the authority and the power to manage other clinicians, while post holders often had insufficient training in management for the task. This led to problems in recruitment to the specialism and a vacuum in local health policy persisted. It was not until the late 1980s that these issues were addressed with the setting up of the Acheson Committee on public health (DHSS, 1988, below).

Prevention and health 1976-1984

In 1976, the Labour government published two consultative documents on health, *Prevention and Health: everybody's business* (DHSS, 1976a) and *Priorities for Health and Personal Social Services in England* (DHSS, 1976b). Though the government was to assert that:

> The publication of *Prevention and Health: Everybody's business*
> represented an unequivocal change of policy within the Health
> Departments towards prevention (DHSS, 1977a, para 12),

the immediate purpose of the document was to stimulate public discussion of the potential and possibilities of prevention (DHSS, 1976a, 1977a). This discussion was to be sustained by the subsequent issuing of papers related to particular subjects: on reducing risk in pregnancy and childbirth (DHSS, 1977b), on 'eating for health' (DHSS, 1979), on 'avoiding heart attacks' (DHSS, 1981a) and on 'drinking sensibly' (DHSS, 1981b). Other contemporary statements and reports, such as the Court Report (DHSS, 1976c) which emphasised the preventive value of child health services, reflected the extent to which the notion of prevention had percolated into health policy discussions.

Three elements of the consultative document on *Prevention and Health* are of particular importance. Firstly, the keynote is one of attention to individual behavioural change. Although, historically, the evidence suggested that the most effective measures for the prevention of disease were those implemented at the level of populations (McKeown, 1979), the document argues that:

> We as a society are becoming increasingly aware of how much
> depends on the attitude and actions of the individual about his
> health... Prevention today is everybody's business (DHSS,
> 1976a, p. 7).

Secondly, all discussion is prefaced by a warning as to the limited availability of resources. The development of preventive policy will be achieved only by the redeployment of existing resources. (1) Thirdly, emphasis is placed on the relationship between prevention and health planning. All three elements are brought out in the paper's closing remarks, which indicate that it:

> will have failed in its purpose if this discussion does not lead in
> turn to positive action to promote health
> * action which individuals take in relation to the health and
> well being of themselves and their family
> * action in planning and reorienting local and national services
> to give a greater emphasis to prevention within whatever
> resources can be made available (DHSS, 1976a, p. 96).

The government's subsequent White Paper (DHSS, 1977a), rather than setting out clear proposals based on the discussion it had itself sought to initiate, represented little more than a cautious reply to the report of an Expenditure Committee inquiry (Expenditure Committee, 1977). Only in its conviction that individuals are responsible for their health did it remain as strident as before. (2) There were no clear plans for government initiatives: action on prevention was expected from Area Health Authorities (AHAs), to whom responsibility for the elaboration and coordination of policy was devolved. Health education and advice-giving to individuals, moreover, was left mainly to the judgement of individual health professionals.

Although the DHSS has repeatedly advocated the sharing of responsibility for prevention between commercial and voluntary organisations, (3) government, the NHS and public bodies (DHSS, 1976b, 1981c, 1988), effective policy responsibility remained diffused rather than shared. The danger in this approach was that because prevention was 'everybody's business' it seemed likely to be nobody's (Expenditure Committee, 1977, para 60). Reports and government statements issued during this period continued to assert that mechanisms of planning and coordination were a key aspect of preventive health policy (Expenditure Committee, 1977; DHSS, 1977a, and note also DHSS, 1988). They referred to a need for collaborative action at ministerial level, and both within the NHS and between the NHS and local authorities.

The reality of the situation, however, was a fragmented structure of administrative agencies at both national and local levels. Policy development was hampered by the organisation of government: issues of preventive policy making cut across the competing interests of ministerial departments. A concern for health expressed by the Department of Health, for example, may be countered by other departments concerned primarily with employment, tax revenue or the interests of producers. This 'departmentalism' or 'departmental pluralism' (Baggott, 1986, 1987) is exacerbated by the strength of departmental allegiances in the British civil service (Baggott, 1991). What may be crucial in getting health issues on the agenda is the position of the health department in relation to others with contrary interests and organisational arrangements. (4) Furthermore, administrative arrangements may restrict not only the formulation of policy but the feasibility of its implementation, too. Fiscal policy, for example, is a relatively simple bureaucratic procedure, while the direct control of production and distribution in the business sector presents much more complex problems to government (Calnan, 1984). (5)

Against this background, the problems of joint planning which arose from the discussion documents of 1976 and 1977 were devolved downward to local agencies to resolve. (6) Yet these authorities themselves had to contend with administrative divisions and a lack of coterminosity in their geographical boundaries (Allsop, 1984; Robertson, 1985; Yarrow, 1986). Although collaboration between health and local authorities had been a key objective of the NHS reorganisation of 1974, local health administration in the period 1974 to 1990 was still divided between District Health Authorities (DHAs, responsible for the management of hospital services) and Family Practitioner Committees (FPCs, which held contracts for general practioner services), and to a lesser extent between health and local authorities. (7) This administrative separation meant the sacrifice of what McLachlan refers to as:

> the potential which may be gained from an organised preventive
> front (McLachlan, introduction to Yarrow, 1986, p. x).

The emphasis on prevention was carried forward in a more or less token way by the *Priorities* documents of 1976 and 1981 (DHSS, 1976b, 1981c) which contain sections on the importance of preventing ill-health. The limitations of the government's approach were revealed by the inquiry into inequalites in health which resulted in the *Black Report* of 1980. (8) In identifying and explaining inequalities, the Report revealed the strong link between poverty and ill-health. Its recommendations sought to redress these by preventing the morbidity and premature mortality of the disadvantaged. In the view of the Report's authors, priority for the preventive services indicated:

> a coherent national programme of enormous scope (Townsend and Davidson, 1982, p. 142).

This was to include the expansion of health education, the regulation of the production and consumption of tobacco, and the extension of screening. The establishment of health and social development programmes was also proposed, which would establish child health clinics and welfare food provision in priority areas. A 'wider strategy' was to be implemented outside the health care system at the heart of which was a comprehensive anti-poverty strategy. A disability allowance and policies for improving family and child health were also mooted. Improvements in working conditions and in housing were seen to be particularly important (Townsend and Davidson, 1982). Appointed by a Labour Secretary of State (David Ennals) in 1977, the Black Report was given short shrift by the new Conservative government on its appearance in 1980 (Townsend and Davidson, 1982). It was cursorily dismissed by the Secretary of State (Patrick Jenkin) on the grounds of its likely cost. Nevertheless, the Report left an indelible mark on health policy discussion by demonstrating the connections between poverty, deprivation and health status.

Prevention played little part in the health policy of the first Thatcher administration of 1979-83. Influenced by the economic and political thought of Friedman and Hayek, the government was unwilling to contemplate planned economic and social intervention. Its ideological commitment to market liberalism was mirrored by its aversion to the Fabianism as represented by the welfare state. It rejected the possibility of rational planning and, with its emphasis on individual choice and freedom, was averse to policies which removed those choices from individuals themselves. The framework of health policy making shifted away from concern with priorities to a more immediate concern with cost and the introduction of management changes into the NHS (DHSS, 1983). Although the NHS itself placed little emphasis on prevention, however, developments in other areas helped to keep prevention and health promotion on the policy agenda.

Alcohol and smoking policy

Smoking, alcoholism, nutrition, dental decay and road traffic accidents were particular concerns of the consultative document of 1976 (DHSS, 1976a). Smoking has been the focus of regulatory legislation, on health grounds, over a long period (see Read, chapt. 6 for a detailed account of policy). The sale of cigarettes to children under 16 was prohibited in 1933, and a ban on cigarette advertising on television introduced in 1964 was extended to radio in 1973. During the 1970s, policies have resulted from negotiations and agreements with the tobacco industry. Cigarette packets now carry health warnings and the scope and quantity of advertising on posters and in sport is restricted. The industry itself has invested in the development of low tar brands. Only since 1983-84 have penal rates of tobacco taxation been used explicitly to discourage smoking (Calnan, 1984, Baggott, 1987).

Alcohol arrived on the policy agenda in the 1960s (Baggott, 1986), although drunkenness and alcoholism tended to be treated separately as issues of public order and mental health respectively. Both judicial and health interests pursued legislation on drinking and driving, bringing about the *Road Safety Act* (1967). While the initial response to alcohol took the form of the provision of clinical services, a shift to prevention was beginning to take place by the late 1970s, promoted by the reports of psychiatric and medical professional bodies (Royal College of Psychiatrists, 1979; Royal College of Physicians, 1980) and government committees. (9) This shift went effectively uncontested, since neither the specialist alcohol treatment units funded in the 1960s nor community services for alcoholics had become well established (Baggott, 1986). In sum, UK governments' approach to policy making intended to reduce smoking and alcohol consumption is perhaps best described as piecemeal (Calnan, 1984, 1989, 1991):

> Government policy in relation to the control of smoking, diet, alcohol and the encouragement of exercise has been characterised by a non-interventionist approach with the emphasis on persuasion and industrial self-regulation ... it is a paternalistic policy which has been based on authoritative knowledge and is inclined towards a more individualist orientation ... (Calnan, 1991, p. 83). (10, 11)

This reluctance to intervene has been explained by commentators as being due to the strength of vested interests and the weakness of those opposing them. Governments' electoral interest and the complex and contradictory motivations produced by competing departmental interests are important associated factors (see, Hann, chapt. 3, Street, chapt. 5 and Read, chapt. 7 for examples). Both the tobacco and alcohol industries in the UK wield considerable economic muscle: in 1984, the drinks industry accounted for 2 per cent of all employment and 5 per cent of GDP (Baggott, 1986). Both lobbies are represented in Parliament through the business and constituency interests of MPs (Calnan, 1984; Taylor, 1984; Baggott, 1986). The voluntary self-regulation of the industries, meanwhile, reflects British policy making style (see, Mills, chapt. 11). It has advantages for business interests in that it makes for stability and allows industry itself a measure of influence. For government, equally, it serves to justify a continued moderate approach as long as it also provides modest concessions (Baggott, 1987, Read, chapt. 6).

Nonetheless, other pressure groups can be seen to have exerted a measure of influence on policy making. Government action on smoking was prompted by a series of reports on *Smoking and Health* produced by the Royal College of Physicians between 1964 and 1983, and by the pressure group ASH (Action on Smoking and Health) established under its auspices in 1971 (Calnan, 1984). The Royal College of Psychiatrists published the similarly influential *Alcohol and Alcoholism* in 1979. While this suggests that the prestige and scientific authority of the medical professions have proved influential enough to turn smoking and, to a lesser extent, alcohol consumption into health political issues, they seem not to have been strong enough to make their recommendations effective (Calnan, 1984). The weak regulation of the production and distribution of food, similarly, can be attributed to inconclusive research findings and a diversity of views within the medical profession (Calnan, 1991). In turn, this points to the extent to which pressure groups of this kind invariably and inevitably face an uphill task. Their achievement lies in working prevention onto the political agenda while industrial lobbies, by contrast, need only to wait and then resist change (Popham, 1981). In addition, in some areas, pressure groups may lack cohesion: the anti-alcohol lobby, for example, has been weakened by conflict between voluntary organisations (Baggott, 1986). (12)

The fact that such activity can change preferences and behaviour can be demonstrated by the diminishing social acceptability of smoking. This has allowed for increasing fiscal intervention by government. Yet governments can lead as well as follow. As Alwyn Smith argues, individual choices do not arise in a vacuum but are influenced by a variety of factors, some of which are a consequence of government policy:

> For example, the national diet has changed profoundly even in the present century. This is simply not an aggregate of individual choices but a reflection of the availability and pricing of foodstuffs and the effects of marketing designed to promote what is profitable to the producers and distributors of food. These in turn are the consequence of political policies governing the use of subsidies and other devices in the pursuit of economic objectives. It would not be a new intrusion on individual liberty for these policies to be guided in the interests of national health (Smith, 1992, p. 377).

Health education

Throughout the 1970s and 1980s, the resort to health education represented a fall-back position for preventive health policy. It accorded well with an emphasis on policies which were relatively inexpensive, immediately practicable, and were in tune with the prevailing ideological and cultural precepts of individual freedom and responsibility. Nevertheless, efforts towards more positive health promotion became an area of significant political tension, the brunt of which was borne by the Health Education Council (HEC). The HEC had been founded in 1968 on the recommendation of a Ministry of Health internal committee, the Cohen committee on health education, which had reported in 1964. (13) It was a public body with independent status and made its first media impact through poster campaigns on smoking and family planning in the early 1970s.

In the early 1980s, the HEC took an independent line. It championed the findings of the Black Report on inequalities in health and lobbied against the tobacco, alcohol and food industries. The Council's Canterbury Report (HEC, 1984) took up the issue of coronary heart disease, calling in particular for increased government regulation of food production and distribution. This was resisted by the Department of Health and Social Security (DHSS) (Ledwith, 1987). The 'emergency topics' of drugs and AIDS then served to heighten the public and political profile of health education (Whitehead,

1987; Baggott, 1991, and Street, chap. 5). (14) In a move designed to make health education work more responsive to the needs of the NHS, the HEC was reconstituted in April 1987 as the Health Education Authority (HEA) responsible directly to ministers. (15) Both sides, however, have acknowledged continued difficulty in defining their relationship (BBC R4, 1991). The government's influence was soon made apparent by the ending of support for community development projects, a number of which had seemed to offer a focus for local health promotion (Beattie, 1991). The Professional and Community Development Division which had been established at the HEA in 1988 was closed in 1989.

Rodmell and Watt (1986) comment that health education in the UK has relied heavily on the medical model of disease:

> Health educators constantly seek affirmation of their activities
> from medical practitioners who retain the power to confer the
> necessary status, but at the same time seek to resist the
> medicalisation which this conferment of status imposes
> (Rodmell and Watt, 1986, p. 3).

As a result, much health education is based on a middle class professional assumption that working class people are best reached through short and simple messages. Farrant and Russell, however, found that working class people wanted more information covering a wider range of evidence which they might then evaluate for themselves (Farrant and Russell, 1987, reported by Calnan, 1991). Thus, despite doubts about its ineffectiveness being shared even by some of those working at the HEC (Beattie, 1991) it has been the individualistic, laissez-faire model of health education which has dominated its work because that has been the approach that has found government support. (16)

As much as the HEC, the HEA has been constrained by governments' sense of political expedience in relation to the threat from vested interests in the business and industrial sector (Farrant and Russell, 1985, 1986, cf Calnan, 1991 and above). Despite, or perhaps even because of, their attempt to widen the agenda for prevention, the work of both bodies has been limited by their dependence on government funding. In this context, government action on health education is compromised to the extent that it is perhaps best described as symbolic. George sums up its weaknesses by suggesting that:

> Government ministers from both sides of the House, along with
> their civil servant advisers, have consistently used the HEC as
> an instant, highly visible, relatively cheap and superficially
> plausible means of responding to pressure to 'do something'
> about a particular health problem ... the quango image and the
> illusion of independence of the HEC allow programmes
> initiated for political reasons to be carried out behind a
> smokescreen of professional and scientific justification (George,
> 1981, p. 51).

Primary care and public health

By the mid-1980s, both general practice and the public health role of community physicians were becoming a focus of policy makers' attention. The Department of Health began to show a new interest in prevention (Klein, 1989), which was supported by a growing concern for the poor health status of the UK population compared to many of its European neighbours and other developed nations (Smith and Jacobson, 1988; NAO, 1989). There was also a surge of interest in health at local level within local government (Moran, 1986) and in individual cities participating in the WHO-sponsored Healthy Cities programme (Ashton and Seymour, 1988). The then Chief Medical Officer (CMO), Donald (now Sir Donald) Acheson also had a particular concern for public health. Meanwhile, in the second half of the 1980s, a number of public health problems came to command media attention. AIDS was the most prominent of these, but others included meningitis, salmonella, legionnaire's disease and the food scares of 1989 and 1990 (17) (see Baggott, 1991). In combination, these factors demanded policy responses in respect of primary care and community physicians in turn.

In 1981, the Royal College of General Practitioners argued that three areas of preventive activity were important in the general practice setting (RCGP, 1981). (18) The individual patient consultation provided an opportunity for screening and health education, while systems could be developed for surveying the practice population and groups at risk. The GP could also liaise with other agencies, such as schools. Some were sceptical of the ability of GPs to carry out this wide variety of roles and suggested that the move towards prevention represented a claim for professional territory (Davies, 1984; Calnan, Boulton and Williams, 1986). In any case, there were a number of obstacles to general practice becoming the focus for illness prevention. First, there was considerable variation between practices in their structure and in their capacity to carry out health promotion. Second, the interest shown in health education by the leaders of the profession was not always shared by the ordinary GP (Calnan, Boulton and Williams, 1986). Third, not all GPs were convinced of the benefits of population screening and health education as the most effective means of prevention (Allsop, 1990).

However, in pursuing a dominant theme of the 1976 *Priorities* document, the government saw health professionals as being the main mediators of health education. They were held to be:

> very well placed to persuade individuals of the importance of
> protecting their health; of the simple steps needed to do so; and
> of accepting that prevention is indeed better than cure (DHSS,
> 1987, para. 1.12).

One of the principal concerns of a new White Paper, *Promoting Better Health* (DHSS, 1987), was to increase the extent of health education and screening in general practice by expanding the primary health care team and encouraging larger practices. Taking up the recommendations of the Cumberlege Report of 1986 (DHSS, 1986), *Promoting Better Health* also emphasised the importance of community nurses' role in health promotion and illness prevention. This increased profile for general practice was encouraged in a number of ways. Greater powers and responsibilities were given Family Practitioner Committees (19) to manage family practitioners. They were given greater control over reimbursing funds for practice improvement and increased flexibility in funding the employment of additional staff. Following the 1990 *NHS and Community Care Act*, incentives were introduced to encourage larger practices to become fundholders in their own right.

New GP contracts were agreed in 1989 (DoH, 1989). General practitioners' terms of service now included requirements to include health promotion and disease prevention within general medical services. The system of remuneration also changed: there was a fee for the clinical assessment of new patients, as well as sessional fees for running health promotion clinics. Further payments were conditional on the achievement of targets for the health screening of elderly people over the age of 75, for the vaccination and immunisation of children, and for cervical cytology. At the same time, however, the government placed new restrictions on the preventive services provided by paramedical professions. It ended free sight testing and introduced charges for dental examination (DHSS, 1987).

By the end of the 1980s, there was evidence of increased activity in general practice. Allsop's (1990) study of facilitators in primary care describes a variety of projects to support change. The Oxford Heart Attack and Stroke Project has been particularly active in developing the role of the practice nurse in screening while, between 1984 and 1988, the numbers of practice nurses doubled from 2000 to 4000 in England and Wales. Fundholding in general practice has also been popular and has led to an extension of services in these practices (Glennerster, Matsaganis and Owens, 1992). Nevertheless, geographical inequalities persist, and practices with poorer facilities tend to be concentrated in certain inner city areas (Leese and Bosanquet, 1989). General practice continues to lack the managerial capability needed to run efficient screening systems. At the same time, too, the constraints of administrative accounting re-emphasise the individualist approach of preventive medicine. It has been suggested that:

> The emphasis on quantifiable behaviour in the White Paper proposals could shift general practitioners from the practice of holistic or socially oriented medicine towards more medically oriented behaviour ... while health promotions and preventions are given importance in 'Promoting better health', these are only measurable as screening and immunization targets and health checks (Bartholomew, 1989, cit Calnan, 1991, p. 197).

Attempting to assess the trends in prevention over the 1980s, McCarthy (1992) shows that there has been an overall decrease in smoking while the take up of cancer screening, general practice health checks and immunisation and vaccination for most childhood diseases has increased. It must be said, however, that both the efficacy of screening in general and its place in general practice have been questioned. Critics argue that it focuses on individual pathology, that it creates a population of 'worried well' and that it incurs high costs with uncertain benefits (Crawford, 1977; McCormick, 1989; Wilkinson, Jones and McBride, 1990; Cribb and Haran, 1991; also see Hann, chapt. 3). There is as yet little clear evidence, for example, that screening reduces deaths from either cancer or coronary heart disease (CHD). While the recent National Audit Office report on CHD suggests that rates are beginning to fall (NAO, 1989), they remain significantly higher than those achieved by the United States and Canada with their more encompassing health promotion programmes (Wells, 1982; McCarthy, 1992).

Meanwhile, a Committee of Inquiry into the Future Development of the Public Health Function, chaired by the Chief Medical Officer Donald Acheson, reported in 1988 (DHSS, 1988). Interestingly, the Committee had been instructed to exclude aspects of public health which were shared by the health department with other government departments. (20) It was told to concentrate narrowly on the role of community physicians and on arrangements for the control of communicable disease. (21) The Committee recommended that Directors of Public Health be appointed in each District Health Authority as 'named leaders of the public health function'. These were to be managerially accountable to the District General Manager. Named responsibility for the control of communicable disease was to be invested by health authorities in a District Control of Infection Officer. While the report of the Acheson Inquiry was accepted in full by the government (Baggott, 1991), the extensive brief accorded to local Directors of Public Health represented a recognition and restatement of problems as much as a plausible solution. The mere renaming of the community medicine specialism seems unlikely to lead to an increase in status either within the medical profession or within health authorities.

The 1990 health service reforms and *The Health of the Nation*

In 1990, the *NHS and Community Care Act* introduced major changes in the organisation of the NHS through the introduction of the internal market. There is now a demarcation between those who purchase health care on behalf of their populations (District Health Authorities or consortia and fundholding GPs) and the Trusts and directly managed units which provide that care. A similar demarcation could well emerge between FHSAs and their GPs. Already in some areas, FHSAs are merging with DHA purchasers to buy community and public health services (Allsop and May, 1992). The implications for public health and the prevention of illness are that it is now the purchasing authorities who assess the health needs of their populations and who determine the importance given to health promotion. As the strategic planning authorities, Regional Health Authorities and the Health Service Management Executive also have a role to play in steering the general direction of health policy at lower levels.

The 1992 White Paper, *The Health of the Nation* (DoH, 1992), provides for the first time a health strategy for England which complements those already published for other parts of the UK. In the context of comparative data on the health status of English regions and between different groups and classes, the document identifies the major causes of illness and deaths before their time and sets priorities and targets. Five key areas for action are identified: heart disease and strokes, cancers, mental illness, sexual health and accidents. Targets are set for percentage decreases in morbidity and mortality for each of these areas. Health authorities and other agencies are expected to adopt policies to achieve these targets within a given time scale.

In the context of the consultations which preceded *The Health of the Nation* two major strategies were identified as important in achieving the goals set by government. The concept of 'health gain' has emerged as a useful tool for agencies to assess which policy or programme to pursue (Welsh Health Planning Forum, 1989). It poses the question of priorities in cost benefit terms: what sorts of investment will make for the greatest benefit in terms of 'adding years to life and life to years'? Looked at in this way, 'health gain' has parallels with the use of QALYs (quality adjusted life years) to compare the costs and benefits of interventions in the hospital sector. Like QALYS, too, notions of 'health gain' appear rational when applied to determining priorities for populations but raise ethical and political problems when they affect individuals (see Honigsbaum, 1991). A second strategy puts emphasis on 'healthy alliances'. In central government, this has taken the form of a Cabinet level committee to coordinate the work of different departments. Within the NHS, the Management Executive has promoted joint working with outside agencies, on the basis that the strategy for health cannot be delivered by the health service alone (NHSME, 1992).

The international context

As suggested in the introduction to this chapter, the UK has lagged behind the countries of North America and Scandinavia in embracing an overall strategy for healthy public policy which is concerned with securing longer lives of better quality for its population. In 1974, for example, Canada published the pioneering *Lalonde Report* (Ministry of National Health and Welfare, 1974) which laid the foundation for healthy public policy. In 1986, the Epp Document (Epp, 1986) outlined strategies for improving health. An emphasis was placed on reducing inequalities, increasing prevention, and enhancing people's capacity to cope with chronic illness and disability. The document went on to put forward three mechanisms to address these challenges: self care, mutual aid and healthy environments. Three structures were proposed to deal with these challenges - fostering public participation, strengthening community health services and inter-sectoral coordination.

Cunningham attributes Canada's success not only to a clearly articulated national strategy but also to a number of other factors (Cunningham, 1991). First, strong public health associations included health professionals, academics and lay people in a shared forum for raising public consciousness while alliances were forged between voluntary organisations in the health field. In Cunningham's view, these associations informed public opinion and allowed government to adopt a radical anti-tobacco policy in the late 1980s. Second, the personal contribution of politicians and public health leaders in government was important. Third, and perhaps most crucial of all, there has been extensive community participation at the local level.

While the US has major problems arising from its method of funding health services, Cunningham nevertheless identifies similar factors which have led to a high profile for public health, albeit in a more patchy way than in Canada (Cunningham 1991). Here too, national objectives were set at federal level over a decade ago, in 1979, with the Surgeon General's report on *Health Promotion and Disease Prevention* (US Public Health Service, 1979). This was followed up in 1990 by *Healthy People 2000* (US Public Health Service, 1990). Other countries have also adopted more or less explicit health promotion strategies. Sweden, for example, is committed to a strategy of health promotion which focuses on the socio-economic conditions of healthy living (Gustafsson and Nettleton, 1992). Norway introduced differential food subsidies in the 1970s to encourage healthy eating (Ringen, 1977; Ziglio, 1986). Interestingly, New Zealand has separated the funding and management of public health services from personal health services in a recently published health strategy, *Your Health and the Public Health* (Ministry of Health, 1991). In contrast, it was not until 1992 that all parts of the UK had published health promotion strategies. At least until then, it seemed reasonable to say that:

> ... even allowing for the complexity of the issues the documents are addressing, the 'strategies' appear as sets of modest, discrete and not terribly well-connected elements which seem likely to provide only partial coverage of the problems they are addressing ... the search for appropriate responses tends to be conducted within the limits set by existing administrative/service   structures   and   responsibilities (Robertson, 1985, p. 209).

Accounting for the underdevelopment of preventive health policy in the UK

The commitment to the prevention of ill-health in the UK has been diluted in a number of ways. First, the New Right ideologies which have dominated the governments of the 1980s, stress a libertarian individualism and the importance of choice. The emphasis has been on informing and educating the individual. Such individualism sits uneasily with the collectivist approach necessary for many aspects of health promotion. Furthermore, governments have been unwilling to acknowledge the relationship between low income, income distribution, (22) unemployment, poor environments and ill-health and have chosen to focus instead on the relationship between life style and health status (Delamothe, 1992), as is witnessed by the fate of the Black Report and its recommendations.

Second, the structure of the NHS and of ministerial government tends to fragment initiatives for collaborative working at both national and local levels. The Department of Health, for example, effectively functions as the Department of the NHS, rather than as a department of health more broadly conceived. As Rudolf Klein has observed, Britain has 'a health policy but no policy for health' (Klein, 1980, cit Baggott, 1991, p. 192). At the local level, as a centrally controlled service with appointed Authorities, the NHS has had difficulty in working with local government and in generating public participation.

Third, prevention is at best tangential to perhaps the most important interest in health policy making, the doctors. Clinicians, almost by definition, have no concern for prevention. General practitioners have made use of a limited conception of prevention in order to define and occupy new areas of professional territory. Public health doctors, meanwhile, have neither been a strong voice within medicine nor an independent one within government.

Fourth, the natural focus of health policy is on health care, not on health promotion, and for significant political reasons:

> The NHS has, by the very fact of its existence, a political constituency: those whose income derives from working in it and those who, as patients, derive some direct benefits from its services. Prevention has no such constituency. Those who will benefit cannot be identified; moreover, the benefit itself is uncertain. For prevention is about the reduction of statistical risk, not about the delivery of certain benefits to specific individuals (Klein, 1989, p. 173).

That is to say that it is precisely because prevention and public health represent a 'political vacuum' (Ledwith, 1987) that this vacuum is unlikely to be filled.

Fifth, and in a rather different way, it may be that it makes little sense to look for genuine commitment to prevention on the part of governments. It is perhaps no coincidence that governments should have taken an interest in prevention in 1976 and in 1991, in the wake of respective reorganisations of the NHS. In each case, governments have used the rhetoric of health education to reassert, if not redefine, the responsibility of individuals for their own health; in this way, they have sought to begin to reduce public expectations both of health services and of health policy making as such. At the same time, prevention also played an important part in redefining the role of GPs according to government as much as to professional interests. It was through prevention that important changes in GPs' conditions of service such as performance targets and fee-for-service payments were introduced and consolidated. In this light, it may be more useful to think of prevention as representing a no more than symbolic goal for policy makers. It has instrumental functions, serving as one way in which relationships between governments, patients and the providers of health care are regulated (Freeman, 1992).

The Health of the Nation: a way forward?

In this context, the publication of *The Health of the Nation* can be seen as step forward. It sets targets which are both a spur to commitment and provide a comparative indicator of progress. It underlines the importance of health education, primary care and collaboration between agencies. At the same time, the *Working for Patients* reforms have also strengthened managerial accountability for the health of populations. Such aims have become part of the mission statements of many commissioning Authorities and Regions and some areas, such as Wales, have demonstrated that progress can be made.

On the minus side, the weaknesses related to administrative structure and political culture remain. Indeed, fragmentation of effort may have been exacerbated by the new managerialism and the introduction of market forces to the NHS (Allsop and May, 1992). The managerialist principles espoused by recent Conservative governments encourage a concentration on core functions while peripheral functions are passed to separate agencies. The proliferation of health service agencies will make collaboration e, not less, difficult while the assessment of health needs and priority setting is one of the most challenging tasks in health care (Osborne and Gaebler, 1992). Market forces, meanwhile, will encourage the Trusts and provider units to concentrate on tangible outputs which can be accurately costed. These factors may make the 'healthy alliances' which Cunningham identified as important in North America much more difficult to achieve. Furthermore, it remains far from clear whether community participation in health policy making can be generated at the local level. Perhaps more fundamentally, the White Paper has done nothing to suggest a change in the political values which underlie the government's health policies. It seems likely that without more radical approaches, greater effort and greater resources, the targets set for five key areas may simply become ends in themselves while the wider aspects of good health are ignored.

Footnotes

1) Indeed, *Prevention and Health* may represent an early variant of the 'nil cost reform'. The joint Secretaries of State, in their foreword, annouce that: 'during the present period of economic constraint it is all the more essential that available resources are used to best effect, bearing in mind that not all preventive measures necessarily require additional, or massive resources' (DHSS, 1976a, p. 7).

2) 'Much ill-health in Britain today arises from over-indulgence and unwise behaviour. Not surprisingly, the greatest potential and perhaps the greatest problem for preventive medicine lies in changing behaviour and attitudes to health' (DHSS, 1977a, para. 131).

3) A number of non-governmental organisations with interests in prevention are listed by Cohen and Moir (1981).

4) Cohen and Henderson (1983) have argued that the inaction resulting from fragmented and vaguely defined responsibilities might be remedied by the appointment of a 'Minister for Prevention'.

5) There is an illuminating parallel here. It has been suggested that legislation in respect of the disabled could only have been produced by means of a Private Member's Bill (Alf Morris's *Chronically Sick and Disabled Persons Act*, 1971). A government initiative could never have borne fruit since so many - up to fourteen - government departments might have been involved (see Boswell and Wingrove, 1974).

6) 'Local initiatives, local decisions and local responsibility are what we want to encourage' (DHSS, 1981a, cit. Hambleton, 1986, p.61).

7) Local authorities retained responsibility for environmental health in 1974. Medical Officers of Environmental Health (MOsEH), who replaced local authorities' Medical Officers of Health (MoSH), were now in fact employed by health authorities but remained managerially accountable to local government.

8) The Report, with a critical introduction describing its virtual suppression by government, was published as Townsend and Davidson (1982).

9) A report on *Alcohol Policies* produced by the government's Central Policy Review Staff in 1979 was widely leaked but not published in the UK (Baggott, 1986).

10) For critical reviews of policy in relation to smoking and tobacco, see Popham (1981), Calnan (1984) and Baggott (1987); in relation to alcohol, Baggott (1986 and 1990); in relation to alcohol and tobacco, see Harrison and Tether (1987) and the collections edited by Maynard and Tether (1990) and Godfrey and Robinson (1990). Alderson's disease-specific focus on the prevention of cancer (Alderson, 1982; see also Doyal and Epstein, 1983) and Calnan on coronary heart disease (Calnan, 1989 and 1991) cover most of the relevant aspects of policy.

11) The flouridation of water supplies in order to prevent dental decay is perhaps the only area where governments and health professionals have consistently urged structural intervention on health grounds (DHSS, 1987; cf. DHSS, 1976a; Expenditure Committee, 1977 and DHSS, 1981d), albeit in a way which does not interfere with markets. Proposals have been resisted by citizens' rights groups and have now been perhaps finally eclipsed by the privatisation of water boards.

12) The level of acrimony was such that the DHSS and the National Council for Voluntary Organisations were moved to conduct a review of the situation which reported in 1982 (NCVO/DHSS, 1982). In 1984, the National Council on Alcoholism, the Federation of Alcoholic Residential Establishments and the Alcohol Education Centre were replaced by the single body Alcohol Concern, which was funded by government (Baggott, 1986).

13) The HEC had a predecessor, the Central Council for Health Education, which had been established in 1927 by the public health doctors' Society of Medical Officers of Health. It was funded by local authorities and voluntary organisations (DHSS, 1988, para. 4.21).

14) Nevertheless, while there is evidence of a marked development of health education in schools, it remains difficult to argue that, before the establishment of the AIDS budget at the HEA, proportionally more funding had been found for health education. The budget of the Health Education Council had remained at roughly 0.1 per cent of NHS hospital spending during the ten years 1977-86 (Whitehead, 1987).

15) A separate Welsh Health Promotion Authority was created at the same time to supercede the former HEC and the Health Education Advisory Committee for Wales. It assumed administrative responsibility for the Welsh AIDS Campaign and for Heartbeat Wales, a regional demonstration project in health promotion launched in 1985.

16) For a critique of the individualism of three specific HEC campaigns, the *Look*

urself! and *Play It Safe!* projects and the *Great British Fun Run* of 1978-1985, see Naidoo (1986).

17) Salmonella in eggs, listeria and bovine spongiform encephalopathy (BSE) in milk and meat.

18) The report seemed concerned 'not to consider in any depth what prevention is or might be but to argue for the essential unity of care and prevention in the work of the GP - and prevention is fashioned very much with this purpose in mind' (Davies, 1984, p.274).

19) FPCs were renamed Family Health Service Authorities (FHSAs) in 1990.

20) 'The Inquiry was instructed to exclude details of those aspects of the public health function which are shared by DHSS with other Government Departments, or are discharged by the Health and Safety Executive (HSE), or the National Radiological Protection Board (NRPB). Nor were we asked to explore the complex social factors underlying health - e.g. housing, employment, poverty - important though we recognise these to be' (DHSS, 1988, para. 1.6).

21) This marks a departure from the pattern of other statements which, since *Prevention and health*, had been predominantly concerned with non-infectious and usually chronic conditions, such as coronary heart disease, the cancers, mental illness and accidental injury; indeed they relate in the first place to what are considered pathogenic aspects of lifestyle such as smoking and drinking, and inadequate eating and habits of exercise. The Acheson Inquiry reflects the resurgent incidence of infectious disease in the 1980s; policy in the 1970s had been more interested in the chronic condition.

22) Wilkinson (1992) has argued, on the basis of a cross-national study of nine developed countries, that standards of health are affected more by the distribution of income within a population than its average level. In other words, making the distribution of income more equal may improve health status.

Bibliography/references

Alderson, M. (ed), (1982), *The Prevention of Cancer*, Edward Arnold, London.

Allsop, J. (1984), *Health Policy and the National Health Service*, Longman, Harlow.

Allsop, J. (1990), *Changing Primary Care: the role of facilitators*, King's Fund Centre, London.

Allsop, J. and May, A. (1992), 'Between the devil and the deep blue sea: managing the NHS in the wake of the 1990 Act', paper prepared for the 22nd Public Administration annual conference, York, England.

Ashton, J. and Seymour, H. (1988), *The New Public Health*, Open University Press, Milton Keynes.

Baggott, R. (1986), 'Alcohol, politics and social policy', *Journal of Social Policy*, vol. 15, no. 4, pp. 467-80.

Baggott, R. (1987), 'Government-industry relations in Britain: the regulation of the tobacco industry', *Policy and Politics*, vol. 15, no. 3, pp. 137-46.

Baggott, R. (1990), *Alcohol, Politics and Social Policy*, Gower, Aldershot.

Baggott, R. (1991), 'Looking forward to the past? The politics of public health', *Journal of Social Policy*, vol. 20, no. 2, pp. 191-213.

Bartholomew, J. E. (1989), *Working for Patients in General Practice*, unpublished MSc dissertation, Royal Holloway and Bedford College, University of London.

BBC R4 (1991), *Face the Facts*, 7 February 1991.

Beattie, A. (1991), 'Knowledge and control in health promotion: a test case for social policy and social theory', in, Gabe, J., Calnan, M. and Bury, M. (eds.), *The Sociology of the Health Service*, Routledge, London.

Boswell, D. M. and Wingrove, J. M. (1974), *The Handicapped Person in the Community. A reader and sourcebook*, Tavistock/Open UP, London.

Calnan, M. (1984), 'The politics of health: the case of smoking control', *Journal of Social Policy*, vol. 13, no. 3, pp. 279-96.

Calnan, M. (1989), 'The politics of preventive medicine: UK government policy and the prevention of coronary heart disease', paper presented to the conference of the Political Studies Association, Warwick.

Calnan, M. (1991), *Preventing Coronary Heart Disease. Prospects, policies and politics*, Routledge, London.

Calnan, M., Boulton, M. and Williams, A. (1986), 'The role of the general practitioner in health education: a critical appraisal', in, Rodmell, S. and Watt, A. (eds.), *The Politics of Health Education. Raising the issues*, Routledge and Kegan Paul, London.

Cohen, D. R. and Henderson, J. (1983), *A Minister for Prevention: an initiative in health policy*, HERU discussion paper 2/83, Health Economics Research Unit, University of Aberdeen, Aberdeen.

Cohen, D. R. and Moir, A. (1981), *Who Does What in Prevention*, HERU discussion paper 09/81, Departments of Community Medicine and Political Economy, University of Aberdeen, Aberdeen.

Crawford, R. (1977), 'You are dangerous to your health: the politics and ideology of victim blaming', *International Journal of Health Services*, vol. 7, no. 4, pp. 663-80.

Cribb, A. and Haran, D. (1991), 'The benefits and ethics of screening for breast cancer', *Journal of the Society of Public Health*, vol. 195, pp. 63-7.

Cunningham, R. (1991), *Promoting Better Health in Canada and the USA: a political perspective*, mimeo, Department of Politics, University of Glasgow, Glasgow.

Davies, C. (1984), 'General practitioners and the pull of prevention', *Sociology of Health and Illness*, vol. 6, pp. 267-89.

Delamothe, T. (1992), 'Poor Britain' (editorial), *British Medical Journal*, vol. 305, pp. 263-4.

DHSS (Department of Health and Social Security) (1976a), *Prevention and Health: everybody's business. A reassessment of public and personal health*, HMSO, London.

DHSS (1976b), *Priorities for Health and Personal Social Services in England. A consultative document*, HMSO, London.

DHSS (1976c), *Fit for the Future. Report of the Committee on Child Health Services, chaired by S D M Court*, vols I and II, cm 6684, HMSO, London.

DHSS (1977a), *Prevention and Health*, session 1977-78, cm 7047, HMSO, London.

DHSS (1977b), *Reducing the Risk: safer pregnancy and childbirth*, HMSO, London.

DHSS (1979), *Eating for Health: a discussion booklet*, HMSO, London.

DHSS (1981a), *Avoiding Heart Attacks*, HMSO, London.

DHSS (1981b), *Drinking Sensibly: a discussion document*, HMSO, London.

DHSS (1981c), *Care in Action: a handbook of policies and priorities for the health and personal social services in England*, HMSO, London.

DHSS (1981d), *Towards Better Dental Health, report of the Dental Strategy Review Group*, HMSO, London.

DHSS (1983), *NHS Management Inquiry (Griffiths Report)*, DA(83)38, DHSS, London.

DHSS (1986), *Neighbourhood Nursing - A Focus for Care. Report of the Community Nursing Review, chaired by Juliet Cumberlege*, HMSO, London.

DHSS (1987), *Promoting Better Health. The government's programme for improving primary health care*, cm 249, HMSO, London.

DHSS (1988), *Public Health in England. The report of the Committee of Inquiry into the future development of the Public Health Function, chaired by Sir Donald Acheson*, cm 289, HMSO, London.

DoH (Department of Health) (1989), *Working for Patients*, cm 555, HMSO, London.

DoH (1991), *The Health of the Nation. A consultative document for health in England*, cm 1523, HMSO, London.

DoH (1992), *The Health of the Nation. A strategy for health in England*, cm 1986, HMSO, London.

Doyal, L. and Epstein, S. S. (1983), *Cancer in Britain. The politics of prevention*, Pluto, London.

Epp, J. (1986), 'National Strategies for Health Promotion', special editorial, *Canadian Journal of Public Health*, July/August, pp. 243-7.

Expenditure Committee (1977), *Preventive Medicine*, first report, session 1976-77, cm 169, HMSO, London.

Farrant, W. and Russell, J. (1985), *HEC Publications: a case study in the production, distribution and use of health information*, final report, Health Education Council, London.

Farrant, W. and Russell, J. (1986), *The Politics of Health Information*, Bedford Way paper 28, Institute of Education, London.

Freeman, R. (1992), *Prevention in Health Policy and the Response to AIDS: a comparative study of the United Kingdom and the Federal Republic of Germany, 1970-1990*, unpublished PhD thesis, University of Manchester, Manchester.

George, D. St. (1981), 'Who pulls the strings at the HEC?', *World Medicine*, 28 November, pp. 51-54.

Glennerster, H., Matsaganis, M. and Owens, P. (1992), *A Foothold for Fundholding*, research report no. 12, Kings Fund Institute, London.

Godfrey, C. and Robinson, D. (eds.), (1990), *Preventing Alcohol and Tobacco Problems*, volume 2, Avebury, Aldershot.

Gustaffson, U. and Nettleton, S. (1992), 'The health of two nations', *International*

Journal of Sociology and Social Policy, vol. 12, no. 3, pp. 1-25.

Hambleton, R. (1986), *Rethinking Policy Planning. A study of planning systems linking central and local government*, University of Bristol School for Advanced Urban Studies, Bristol.

Harrison, L. and Tether, P. (1987), 'The co-ordination of UK policy on alcohol and tobacco: the significance of organisational networks', *Policy and Politics*, vol. 15, no. 2, pp. 77-90.

HEC (Health Education Council) (1984), *Coronary Heart Disease Prevention. Plans for Action*, a report based on an interdisciplinary workshop conference held at Canterbury on 28-30 September 1983, Pitman/HEC, London.

Honigsbaum, F. (1991), *Who Shall Live? Who Shall Die? Oregon's health financing proposals*, King's Fund College Papers 4, King's Fund College, London.

Klein, R. (1980), 'Between nihilism and utopia in health care', lecture given at Yale University, September.

Klein, R. (1989), *The Politics of the NHS*, second edition, Longman, Harlow.

Ledwith, F. (1987), 'Lest we forget the common good', *Health Service Journal*, 30 April, pp. 500-1.

Leese, B. and Bosanquet, N. (1989), 'High and low incomes in general practice', *British Medical Journal*, vol. 298, pp. 932-4.

Lewis, J. (1986), *What Price Community Medicine?*, Wheatsheaf, Brighton.

McCarthy, M. (1992), 'Preventive medicine and health promotion', in, Beck, E., Lonsdale, S., Newman, S. and Patterson, D. (eds.), *In the Best of Health? The status and future of health care in the UK*, Chapman Hall, London.

McCormick, J. (1989), 'Cervical smears: a questionable practice', *The Lancet*, vol. 22, p. 207.

McKeown, T. (1979), *The Role of Medicine: dream, mirage or nemesis?*, Blackwell, Oxford.

Maynard, A. and Tether, P. (eds.), (1990), *Preventing Alcohol and Tobacco Problems*, volume 1, Avebury, Aldershot.

Ministry of Health (NZ) (1991), *Your Health and the Public Health*, Ministry of Health, Wellington.

Ministry of National Health and Welfare (Canada) (1974), *A New Perspective on the Health of Canadians (the Lalonde Report)*, Government of Canada, Ottawa.

Moran, G. (1986), 'Health promotion in local government: a British experience', *Health Promotion*, vol.1, no. 2, pp. 191-200.

Naidoo, J. (1986), 'Limits to Individualism', in, Rodmell, S. and Watt, A. (eds.), *The Politics of Health Education. Raising the issues*, Routledge and Kegan Paul, London.

NCVO (National Council for Voluntary Organisations)/DHSS (1982), *Voluntary Organisations in Alcohol Misuse*, DHSS, London.

NAO (National Audit Office) (1989), *Report of the Comptroller and Auditor General: NHS coronary health*, HMSO, London.

NHSME (National Health Service Management Executive) (1992), *The Health of the Nation: healthy alliances, working together*, NHSME, Leeds.

OHE (Office of Health Economics) (1992), *Compendium of Health Statistics for 1992*, Office of Health Economics, London.

Osborne, D. and Gaebler, T. (1992), *Reinventing Government*, Addison Wesley,

Massachusetts.

Popham, G. (1981), 'Government and smoking: policy making and pressure groups', *Policy and Politics*, vol. 9, no. 3, pp. 331-47.

Ringen, K. (1977), 'The case of Norway's nutrition and food policy', *Social Science and Medicine*, vol. 13C, pp. 33-41.

RCGP (Royal College of General Practitioners) (1981), *Health and Prevention in Primary Care*, Royal College of General Practitioners, London.

Robertson, A. (1985), 'Trends in health policy: lessons from an international perspective', *in*, McCrone, D. (ed.), *The Scottish Government Yearbook 1985*, Unit for the Study of Government in Scotland, Edinburgh.

Rodmell, S. and Watt, A. (eds.), (1986), *The Politics of Health Education. Raising the issues*, Routledge and Kegan Paul, London.

Royal College of Physicians (1980), *A Recommendation for the Prevention of Alcohol-Related Disorders*, Royal College of Physicians, London.

Royal College of Psychiatrists (1979), *Alcohol and Alcoholism*, Tavistock, London.

Smith, A. (1992), 'Setting a strategy for health', *British Medical Journal*, vol. 304, pp. 376-8.

Smith, A. and Jacobson, B. (1988), *The Nation's Health: a strategy for the 1990s*, report of an independent steering committee, King's Fund, London.

Taylor, R. C. R. (1984), 'State intervention in postwar western European health care: the case of prevention in Britain and Italy', in, Bornstein, S., Held, D. and Krieger, J. (eds.), *The State in Capitalist Europe*, George Allen and Unwin, London.

Townsend, P. and Davidson, N. (1982), *Inequalities in Health. The Black Report*, Penguin, Harmondsworth.

US Public Health Service (1979), *Healthy People. The Surgeon General's report on health promotion and disease prevention*, US Department of Health and Human Services, Washington DC.

US Public Health Service (1990), *Healthy People 2000*, US Department of Health and Human Services, Washington DC.

Wells, N. (1982), *Coronary Heart Disease: the scope for prevention*, Office of Health Economics, London.

Welsh Health Planning Forum (1989), *Strategic Intent and Directions for the NHS in Wales*, NHS Directorate, Welsh Office, Cardiff.

Whitehead, M. (1987), *The Health Divide: inequalities in health in the 1980s*, Health Education Council, London.

Wilkinson, C., Jones, C., and McBride, J. (1990), 'Anxiety caused by abnormal results of a cervical smear test: a controlled trial', *British Medical Journal*, vol. 300, p. 440.

Wilkinson, R. (1992), 'Income distribution and life expectancy', *British Medical Journal*, vol. 304, pp. 165-8.

Yarrow, A. (1986), *Politics, Society and Preventive Medicine. A review*, Nuffield Provincial Hospitals Trust, London.

Ziglio, E. (1986), 'Uncertainty in health promotion: nutrition policy in two countries', *Health Promotion*, vol. 1, no. 3, pp. 257-68.

Acknowledgements

Richard Freeman is grateful to the Economic and Social Research Council for funding the doctoral research on which part of this paper is based.

3 The decision to screen

Alison Hann

In Britain, as in most other Western European countries, breast cancer is the most common cancer in women, accounting for 20 per cent of all female cancer deaths. Each year, in the UK, 24,000 women are diagnosed as having cancer of the breast, and about 15,000 will sadly die as a result. Nationally, over the last ten years, there has been a slight increase both in the number of cases and in the number of deaths. Britain is in the unenviable position of having the highest breast cancer mortality rate in the whole world (World Health Statistics Annual, 1985; Cancer Research Campaign Factsheet 6, 1988)

Although the causes of breast cancer are not known at the present time, there is some evidence to suggest that certain groups of women are at a slightly higher risk of developing the disease than others. Unlike cervical cancer, which occurs mainly in women of social class five and six, breast cancer is more common among women of social classes one and two. There also seems to be a link with a woman's reproductive history. For example, a woman who has her first pregnancy before the age of 20 is in a slightly lower risk group than a woman who postpones motherhood until after 25 or has no children at all. There also appears to be a link between early menarche and the risk of breast cancer. But, despite these 'high risk' factors, only a minority of women with breast cancer display known high risk factors. It is therefore very difficult to pin point those women who are likely to develop breast cancer with any great accuracy.

Once the disease has been accurately diagnosed, there is little consensus about how the disease should be managed, and what treatment there is, seems not to significantly effect the survival rates. For example there has been an on-going controversy concerning the usefulness of radical breast surgery after cancer diagnosis (as opposed to more conservative surgery coupled with chemotherapy). Both sides in the debate claiming that the other method of breast cancer management is irresponsible and causes more harm than good.

However, it has long been assumed by some (though by no means all) doctors and surgeons that early detection of breast cancer at a pre-clinical stage would improve the prognosis of any woman with breast cancer. Although 90 per cent of breast lumps were found by the woman herself, by the time she presented, the cancer would be at a fairly advanced state and the prognosis would be poor. It was felt that some method of detecting cancers at an earlier stage would be an effective way of reducing the mortality rate of women with breast cancer. It was with this in mind that in 1985 an educational programme was initiated by community health departments, family planning clinics and general practitioners (GPs) which would teach women how to examine their breasts for very small lumps. This was despite the fact that results from clinical trials into the effectiveness of breast self-examination (BSE) were inconclusive (Hill 1988; Davey, 1970; Hobbs, 1985; Hill, 1988). However, there was an alternative to BSE - breast cancer screening by mammography. There had been several overseas trials, most of which looked promising, and several European countries had begun national breast cancer screening programmes, in the hopes of reducing the mortality rates (e.g. Sweden). Screening by mammography was very much on the medical agenda but, unlike cervical cancer, it had not yet appeared on the political agenda.

On the 2nd of July, 1985, breast cancer screening apparently jumped onto the political agenda. Mr Clarke, the then Minister for Health, announced in the House of Commons that he had asked Professor Sir Patrick Forrest to chair a working group which would examine the information available in support of breast cancer screening by mammography. The decision to set up a working group had apparently been taken as a response to the results of a recently published study carried out in Sweden, which the Minister claimed had: 'removed many of the doubts previously attached to the value of mammographic screening for breast cancer'(HC Debates, 1987, p. 272, 25 February).

The Forrest Report

The working group's terms of reference were:

1) To consider the information now available on breast cancer screening by mammography; the extent to which this suggests necessary changes in UK policy on the provision of mammographic facilities and the screening of symptomless women, and

2) To suggest a range of policy options and assess the benefits and costs associated with them; and set out the service planning, manpower financial and other implications of implementing such options (HC Debates, 1987, p. 272, 25 February).

The Forrest Committee duly published an interim report in January 1986, with the full report being published in November of the same year. The conclusions of the interim report were that:

> The information already available from principal overseas trials led us to conclude that deaths from breast cancer in women aged 50-64 years who are offered screening by mammography can be reduced by one third or more (HC Debates, 1987, p. 272, 25 February).

In the final report, the committee made more detailed recommendations. These were that:

1) Breast cancer screening with mammography should be implemented on a nation-wide basis for the screening of symptomless women (or at least those aged between 50 and 64).

2) Pilot centres should be set up to monitor and confirm the findings of the working group. The results of the UK trial, (which was due to publish in 1988) would provide vital epidemiological evidence that the proposed nation-wide programme would replicate the findings of the overseas controlled trials.

3) One view mammography was sufficient to significantly reduce the mortality rate from breast cancer.

4) The screening interval should be three years.

5) Suggestions were made concerning the administration of the screening procedure, i.e. how women were to be invited to attend for screening, the call and recall system, how abnormalities once found should be dealt with by the administrative machinery.

6) Cost benefit appraisals, manpower calculations and the implications for the National Health Service (NHS).

Forrest recommended that the basic mammographic screen should be performed either in a static screening unit or, in more rural areas, in a custom-made mobile screening unit. Each breast screening unit would serve the needs of approximately 10,000 women in the target population each year. It was recognised that the basic screen could only separate those women who had an 'abnormality' from those women who did not, and a number of women would have 'inadequate films'. Quality assurance was therefore most important if the sensitivity of mammograms was to be maintained at a high standard. After screening, there would be an assessment of those women who had been identified as having an abnormality. Such assessment could include a further mammogram (two view this time), clinical breast examination, ultrasonograph, fine-needle aspiration or biopsy.

The recommendations that the Forrest Committee made in the interim report were essentially the same as those made in the final report ten months later. However, despite the positive findings of the interim report, the government did not immediately respond by implementing the recommendations. It was not until February 1987, a year after the publication of the interim report (and three months before the general election), that the Secretary of State for Social Services, Norman Fowler, announced the intention to implement Forrest:

> The Government accept the proposals made in the report and accordingly have decided to implement a national breast cancer screening service (HC Debates, 1987, p. 272, 25 February).

The announcement of the implementation of the Forrest Committee's recommendations, however, were not met with universal praise. Mr Fowler was attacked by several members of the House. Michael Meacher asked if the Secretary of State was aware that: 'this was a grossly inadequate response to the Forrest report, when 5,000 women have died of breast cancer while the Government have been sitting on the report since last year?' In reply to this Mr. Fowler said that: 'That is a disappointing and grudging response'. However, while some thought that the government's response to the Forrest report was inadequate, (too little, too late), there were few voices raised against the idea of a national programme of screening for breast cancer. What doubts there were tended to be expressed in medical journals and not in the public arena. Others were pleased and relieved that the government had provided money to set the programme up. (Previously, the Government had directed health authorities to computerise call and recall systems for cervical cancer tests without providing any central funding). It was recognised that the programme would be expensive to launch, as many hospitals would need to build new units, buy new equipment and employ extra staff. Each regional health authority was funded according to the number of women who were living in the area. For every half a million women, the region would receive £150,000, together with £206,000 yearly revenue. Exactly how the money was spent was a matter of negotiation between the programme manager and the health authority, but the important point was that the money was to be 'ring-fenced'. Most breast screening units were to have a programme manager, a budget holder, screening staff, office staff and a management team, although some units were organised slightly differently. An advisory committee was set up to monitor the efficiency and effectiveness of the breast screening service nationally.

However, although breast cancer screening had not apparently been a political issue prior to the statement in the House in 1985, it would be a mistake to assume that it had not been an issue within the medical world. Indeed, Forrest had been investigating the viability of screening for breast cancer using mammography prior to the setting up of the working group. And in fact we need to go back at least this far to understand the process which led up to the decision to implement the Forrest Report.

The policy network

In 1978, a committee was set up by the Department of Health and Social Security (DHSS) to consider how breast cancer screening might be developed in Britain. The aim was to establish a randomised trial of screening using several different methods, e.g. mammography, BSE and clinical breast examination (CBE). The trial was intended to last for seven   years. The committee consisted of 41 members, 15 of whom were later to serve in some capacity on the Forrest Committee (including Forrest himself).   The group were hoping to replicate the findings of the Health Insurance Plan (HIP) of Greater New York (1963-66) trial which had published its findings in 1971.   It was assumed by most observers that if the HIP findings were replicated the results would favour the setting up of some sort of screening service.

Outside medical circles, pressure was growing.   Both the Women's National Commission (WNC) and the National Council of Women were bringing pressure to bear on government departments to implement some sort of national breast cancer screening programme.   The WNC is an advisory committee to government whose remit is to ensure by all possible means that the informed opinions of women are given their due weight in the deliberations of government. (1)

In November of 1983, the WNC published a report on *Women and the Health Service*, in which it urged the government to implement the findings of the UK trial currently in progress (Women's National Commission, 1985).   At the time the report was published the government Co-Chair of the WNC was Mrs. Edwina Currie, who was actively supporting moves towards the setting up of a breast cancer screening programme. At the same time, the National Council of Women were also actively advocating the implementation of some form of national breast cancer screening.   Both these organisations feel they were instrumental in the setting up of the Forrest Committee.

But, although there seemed to be a high level of consensus within the policy network, it must not be forgotten that the controversy continued within medicine.

The technical debate

By the time the Forrest Committee was created there had been some ten or more studies completed into screening for breast cancer, although not all of these used mammography as the single modality. The Forrest Committee chose to use evidence from two of the completed trials (the HIP trial in America and the 'Two Counties' trial in Sweden), it also used evidence from the UK trial even though this trial was incomplete and its findings, at that time, unpublished. The use of this evidence by the Forrest Committee, and indeed the evidence from all but one of the overseas trials using mammography as a screening modality, has been severely criticised. Doubts have been raised in medical circles as to the usefulness of breast cancer screening using the mammogram and therefore the wisdom of implementing a national programme based on equivocal evidence. The purpose of this section is to outline, very briefly, the major studies of breast cancer screening using mammography and the controversy that surrounds them.

One of the earliest, and most widely quoted clinical trials, was the HIP trial that was started in New York in 1963. The trial led the authors of the report to conclude that there were grounds for 'cautious optimism' (Shapiro et al., 1971). The study compares the experience of a random sample of 31,000 women, aged between 40 -60 years. Some critics of the study have said that the authors of the report were quite right to be cautious. One critic, Petr Skrabanek, points out that:

Less than 20 per cent of the newly diagnosed cases were detected by mammography before they could have been detected by palpation. It has been estimated that only six deaths from breast cancer in seven years in a study involving 60,000 women could have been prevented by including mammography (Skrabanek,1989).

However, the follow up trial for the HIP study produced slightly more positive results. They were able to claim a 30 per cent reduction in mortality from breast cancer during the first ten years of follow up in the total group of study women aged 40-60 at entry. By the end of 18 years from entry, the reduction was about 25 per cent and the authors claimed that: 'Mammography was an important contributor to this reduction in mortality' (Andersson et. al., 1988).

However, it has been suggested that, due to the design of the HIP study, it is very difficult to isolate the effect that mammography had on the reduction in mortality.

In 1974, there was another controlled trial, this time in the Netherlands. The main aim of this study was to test the effectiveness of screening using mammography but also, and perhaps more importantly, to test the oestrogen window hypothesis, exploring the links between oestrogen and women's menstrual cycle and the development of breast cancer. Two follow up studies were carried out, the DOM II in 1981, and the DOM III in 1982. The results from these trials were disappointing. In the initial screening round, 17 breast cancers were detected for every 45,388 women years - a rate of 0.4 per 1,000. This does improve though, until at eight years after the first screening the number of detections is 4.0 per 1,343 women years, which is 3.0 per thousand. But it became evident that although small cancers were detected, there were still many that were node positive, that is, if cancer cells were detected in the lymph nodes: 'Detecting more small cancers did not increase the (relative) number of cancers with negative axilliary nodes' (De Ward et al., 1974). The authors also concluded that: 'the screening of women younger than 50 years old does not give promising results'. The Nijmegen trial in 1975, which was a breast cancer screening trial using mammography every two years, found that the breast cancer screening had caused no drop in mortality rates at all. The authors were forced to conclude that: 'Early treatment of breast cancer may not influence the chance of recovery, but may merely postpone the death due to breast cancer' (Verbeek et al., 1984).

The authors also recognised the problems associated with false negatives, two thirds of which are due to technical reasons, but one third of which were due to fast growing tumours that are undetected at the time of screening.

This was not the only trial which failed to reach a positive conclusion about the effectiveness of breast cancer screening using mammography. The Malmo trial, which started in 1976, reached the cautious conclusion that mammographic screening *may* lead to reduced mortality from breast cancer, at least in women aged 55 or over.

But the study which has been most widely quoted, both by supporters of the breast cancer screening lobby and its opponents is the Swedish trial. This trial was started in 1977. It was designed to investigate the efficacy of mass screening with single view mammography in reducing mortality from breast cancer. 162,981 women aged 40 or over, and who were living in the two counties of Kopparberg and Ostergotland, were enrolled in the study. Each woman in the study group was offered screening every two or three years depending on age. Women in the control group were not offered screening. The authors claimed that in women aged between 40 and 74 years, there was a 31 per cent reduction in mortality. This study was one of the studies used by the Forrest Committee during its deliberations, and it is therefore worth looking in some detail at the criticisms of the trial.

Petr Skrabanek outlines the main areas of criticism:

> The Swedish study has raised more questions than it has solved. The design of the study is unclear ... The Lancet paper provided no information on interval cancers and no overall mortality. Although the authors noted a 30 per cent to 40 per cent excess of breast cancers in the study group, which suggests overdiagnosis and overtreatment, it appears that the overall mortality in the study group was slightly higher than in the control group; not a single life was saved in more than half a million women years ... As the cause of death was not ascertained by independent pathologists, it might be more reliable to compare all deaths in breast cancer cases regardless of ascription on the death certificate. Viewed in this light, the benefit to screened women is dramatically reduced, and in the Ostergotland limb of the trial, is non-existent (Skrabanek, 1988).

The 30 per cent reduction in mortality rates was the same as that reported by the researcher conducting the HIP trial, despite the fact that the compliance rate in Sweden was twice as good and the mammographic equipment was much more sophisticated. In absolute terms, the 30 per cent reduction was 40 deaths less in 78,000 women screened in eight years. That is, one death less per 10,000 women years. This is more than off-set by about 100 more deaths in the screened group from other causes.

The next three major trials, The Canadian Trial, (Miller, 1986, the BCCP trial (Baker, 1982, and the UK trial (Chamberlain, 1989), all failed to report significant positive findings. The conclusion of the researchers on the Canadian project was that: '... breast cancer screening requires continued evaluation and cannot currently be adopted as a population manoeuvre' (Miller, 1986). Furthermore they point out that assumptions made about the usefulness of improvements in technology, may be wrong. They certainly make it clear that the fact that breast lumps can be detected earlier does not necessarily mean an improvement in terms of mortality reduction.

Summary of the objections

Opponents of the national breast cancer screening programme, and of the Forrest report, object on the following grounds:

1) Mammography is not a good screening test, since its positive predictive value in asymptomatic populations is low (Skrabanek, 1989). Skrabenek maintains that: 'The implementation of the Forrest report, would result in over 100,000 mammograms a

year showing false positive results'. Also, mammography is not sensitive enough, that is, it can miss even quite large cancers: '... in a recent series of 139 palpable tumours in women under the age of 51, 44 per cent were false negatives' (Skrabanek, 1989). The high levels of false positives mean that many women will be called back for assessment, and this can cause high levels of anxiety both in the women concerned, and their families.   If women have been diagnosed as having an abnormality by a private screening service they are 'fed' back into the NHS for assessment, and that can cause considerable delay between the abnormality being found and the patient receiving either reassurance or treatment (Fentman, 1988). The overdiagnosis caused by the high number of false positives also causes unnecessary biopsies, and sometimes unnecessary breast surgery.   There has been some suggestion that repeated exposure to low dose radiation can cause breast cancer (Modan et al., 1989).

2) The decision to implement the Forrest recommendations was premature.   The results of the UK trial were not known.   What was the point of setting up a randomised trial if the results were irrelevant?   Also, there has been substantial criticism of the evidence from the overseas trials that have used mammography to screen for breast cancer (Ellman, 1987; Radway, 1988; Reidy, 1988).

3) The interval between screening rounds is too long, and one view mammography is insufficient.

4) The evidence that detection of breast cancer at an earlier stage improves the prognosis is not conclusive.

5) It is not ethical. This last objection is one made by Skrabenek, who believes that (a) women should not be included in clinical trials without their full knowledge and consent (Skrabanek, 1988), (b) women should not be encouraged to carry out BSE as it has not been proved to be of any benefit at all, (Skrabanek, 1988; Wright,1986; Forrest Report, 1986; Frank, 1985; Day and Miller, 1986; Dowle et al., 1987; Hill, 1988; Hobbs, 1985):

> Yet, as with other unproved preventive measures, cancer societies as well as other well meaning but misguided groups are allowed freely to broadcast misleading propaganda. Breast cancer screening recommendations were described by one editorialist as 'a confusing mixture of half truths, unsupported by medical evidence to date, which only adds to the anxiety and uncertainty that always seems to cloud rational discussion of what knowledge we do - or especially do not have - about breast cancer' (Skrabanek, 1990).

6) Breast cancer screening using mammography is expensive, time consuming and difficult. The money would be more productively used if it were spent on researching into the underlying causes of cancer.
    So, why was the national breast cancer screening programme implemented given how equivocal the scientific evidence seems to be?

Why was Forrest implemented?

The first time that breast cancer was mentioned as a political issue in the House of Commons was on the 2nd of July 1985. It would be misleading though to assume that breast cancer and breast cancer screening had not been an issue at all prior to this. For example, in March 1978 a national breast cancer service was called for at the Trades Union Congress Women's Conference. Other women's groups, such as the Royal College of Nursing (RCN), were pressing strongly for the government to at least investigate the feasibility of a national breast cancer screening programme, especially since the published results of the Swedish study had been so encouraging. But as we have seen, not all of the experts were agreed that breast cancer screening, if it were implemented on a national scale, would necessarily be desirable. The main thrust of the objections, in the early stages, were based on the cost of the service to the NHS. For example, *The Times* reported on 19 July, 1978, that:

> At present there seems little prospect of mass screening being offered by the Health Service to all women in Britain, even those over the age of 50. Use of the simplest screening methods seems unlikely to bring the cost below £5 for each woman screened.

A similar worry was expressed in another article in *The Times* seven years later when Nicholas Timmins produced an estimate of the cost of finding a single case of breast cancer: '... on this basis it costs £80,000 to detect a single case of breast cancer because the chances of a case being discovered by screening are 1 in 500'.

But these sorts of criticism were few and far between, those who said anything at all, were largely in favour of breast cancer screening. Some groups had a higher profile than others.

The RCN, the Women's National Cancer Campaign, The Women's National Commission, the National Council of Women and the women's section of the TUC were all pressing very strongly for government action over breast cancer screening, as were several Labour MPs, including Clare Short, and the first minister for women's health, Edwina Currie.

The Royal College of Nursing commented in a press conference that:

> Further delay on the pretext of waiting for the results of yet more research is more prevarication at the expense of women's lives, and there are fears that ministers may decide to pump a few millions into mammography as a pre-election gesture without giving sufficient thought to the service that is needed.

Pressure from these groups increased as the government appeared to do nothing after the publication of the Forrest Report. Dr. Barbara Thomas, clinical director of the Jarvis Centre, said that women should make loud and persistent demands to get the government to take action:

> If we can get any woman in the cancer range who notices a change to demand a mammogram we will have achieved something. If they can't get one, they should write to their MPs. The campaign by women to introduce cervical cancer screening paid off. Women should now be demanding the same for breast cancer.

But the various women's groups were not the only people applying pressure. Members of the Forrest Committee were becoming very frustrated at the apparent lack of government action after the publication of the report and they were supported by the Cancer Control Campaign who felt that the government was dragging its feet. One member of the Forrest Committee remarked to me that the feeling of the committee at the time was that ministers were sitting on the report because the did not like the conclusions and recommendations that the committee had made, and were therefore intending to ignore it.

It is clear, then, from all of the above evidence that groundswell opinion was certainly in favour of a national breast cancer screening service, and there were a considerable number of influential groups and individuals who were pressing for it. That is not to say that all of these groups were 'informed' in the sense that they may not have been fully aware of the medical controversy surrounding mammography as a screening modality. Indeed it appears that some groups were not concerned with the medical debate at all but saw screening as something which, by definition, ought to be of benefit to women in general and were anxious to exert pressure on that basis. To some extent this is still the case, with some women's groups still pressing for the routine screening of women under the age of 50, even though there is overwhelming evidence that screening women in this age group is not beneficial. One reason for this, I think, is that the issue of breast cancer has gained an increasingly high media profile. Most women are aware that breast cancer is (a) on the increase in Britain, and (b) often results in the loss of a breast or, all too often, loss of life. For these reasons the control of breast cancer (through whatever means), and improving the prognosis of women who have contracted the disease, are issues that are emotionally highly charged. Because the issue of breast cancer is so emotive, many groups appear to have distanced themselves both from the medical discourse on the subject and also the problems raised by resource allocation. But pressure of this kind, although hard to ignore, is not impossible to ignore, and it is not my opinion that this pressure alone was responsible for the government's decision to implement Forrest. Another element needs to be added to the equation, and I think that this can be found by looking at the consensus generated by the medical experts who were involved in the various committees and research projects. A number of individuals who were closely involved with the Forrest Committee were also involved in the advisory committees to the DHSS, the UK trial and the BCTS (British Cancer Trials Coordinating Sub-Committee). This network of experts who had been involved with breast cancer screening in various ways for a number of years, formed a formidable lobby which used an impressive amount of medical evidence to back up its demands. These two elements (the 'lay' pressure and the professional pressure), together also with the media attention and the growing awareness that breast cancer was responsible for an increasing number of women's deaths, meant that the government was in a position where something highly visible needed to be done to diffuse mounting criticism. And it must not be forgotten that the general election of 1987 was fast approaching. The announcement therefore of the government's intention to implement Forrest coupled, as it was, with promises to increase funding into AIDS research provided the ideal solution to the government's dilemma, and provided it with a not inconsiderable helping of political capital as well.

Footnote

1) The origins of the commission lie in a body known as the Women's Consultative Council, which was set up in 1962, to keep the government of the day (Harold Macmillan's) 'in touch with women's thinking'. Under Harold Wilson the group was revamped and given more specific terms of reference. Today the WNC has 50 member organisations and 20 associate member organisations. The current government Co-Chairperson is Baroness Denton, and her elected colleague is Mrs. Margaret Morrison, former president of the Civil Service Union. In 1986, a Ministerial Group on Women's Issues was formed. This group is chaired by a Home Office Minister and the WNC's government Co-Chairperson is its vice-chair.

Bibliography/references

Andersson, A. (et al.) (1988), 'Mammographic Screening and Mortality From Breast
    Cancer: The Malmo Mammographic Trial', *British Medical Journal*, vol. 279,
    pp. 943-8, 15 October.
Baker, E. (et al.) (1982), 'Breast Cancer Reduction Demonstration Project: Five Year
    Summary Report', *Cancer*, vol. 32, 194.
Bunker, C. and Baum, M. (eds) (1989), 'Mass Mammography - The Time For
    Reappraisal - Technology and Surgical Policy', *International Journal of
    Technology Assessment in Health Care*, Special Issue, Spring.
Cancer Research Campaign (1988), 'Factsheet 6'.
Chamberlain, J. (et al.) (1989), 'First Results In Mortality Reduction in the UK. Trial
    of Early Detection of Breast Cancer', *The Lancet*, vol. 2, 29 August.
Davey, J.B., Greening, W.P. and Makella, J.A. (1970), 'Is Screening for Cancer
    Worthwhile?, *British Medical Journal*, vol. 3, pp. 696-9, 19 September.
Day, M. and Miller, A.B. (1986), *Canadian National Breast Screening Study:
    Screening for Breast Cancer*, Hans Huber Publishers, Toronto.
Department of Health and Social Security (DHSS), *Breast Cancer Screening*, Report
    to the Health Ministers of England and Wales by a Working Group Chaired by
    Sir Patrick Forrest, HMSO, London.
De Ward, F., Collette, H. (et al.) (1974), 'The DOM Project for the Early Detection
    Of Breast Cancer', *The Lancet*, vol. 1, pp. 1224-6.
Dixon, T. (1987), 'Breast Cancer: The Debate Continues', *Canadian Family
    Physician*, vol. 33, pp. 317-8.
Dowle, C. S. and Blamey, R. (et al.) (1987), 'Preliminary Results of the Nottingham
    Breast Self Examination Education Programme', *British Journal of Surgery*,

vol. 174.

Dowle, C.S., Mitchell, A. (et al.) (1987), 'Preliminary Results of the Nottingham Breast Self-Examination Education Programme', *British Journal of Surgery*, vol. 74.

Ellman, R. (1987), 'A Cautious Two Cheers for Screening', *Preventive Medicine*, February, p. 3.

Fentman, I. (1988), 'Pensive Women, Painful Vigils', *The Lancet*, vol. 1, pp. 1041-2, 7 May.

Frank, A. (1985), 'Breast Self-Examination, More Harm than Good?', *The Lancet*, vol. 2, pp. 654-7.

Hill, D. (1988), 'Self-examination of the Breast, Is It Beneficial?', *British Medical Journal*, vol. 297, 23 July.

Hobbs, P. (1985), 'The Use of Breast Self-Examination as a Screening Modality', *Journal of the Institute of Health Education*, vol. 23, part 4, pp. 125-133.

Miller, A. (1980), 'The Canadian National Breast Cancer Screening Study', *Clinical Investigative Medicine*, vol. 4, pp. 227-58.

Modan, B., Cherit, A., Alfandary, E., and Katz, L. (1989), 'Increased Risk of Breast Cancer After Low Dose Irradiation', *The Lancet*, vol. 1, pp. 629-74, 25 March.

Radway, A. (1988), 'Breast Cancer Screening, a Continuous Controversy', *Cancer Topics*, vol. 7, no. 2, September/October.

'Recent Trends in Breast Surgery in the United Kingdom',(1986), *British Medical Journal*, vol. 292, 7 June.

Reidy, J. (1988), 'Controversy over Mammographic Screening', *British Medical Journal*, vol. 297, 15 October.

Shapiro, S. (et al.) (1971), 'Periodic Breast Cancer Screening in Reducing Mortality From Breast Cancer', *Journal of the American Medical Association*, vol. 215, no. 11, 15 March.

Skrabanek, P. (1988), 'The Physician's Responsibility to the Patient', *The Lancet*, vol. 1, pp. 1155-6, 21 May.

Skrabanek, P. (1988), 'The Benefits of Mass Screening Rests on Equivocal Evidence', *Diagnostic Imaging International*, vol. 4, no. 3, June.

Skrabanek, P. (1988), 'Breast Cancer Screening - a UK Showdown', *British Journal of Hospital Medicine*, 18 October.

Skrabanek, P. (1989), 'Shadows Over Mammography', *Clinical Radiology*, vol. 40.

Skrabanek, P. (1990), 'Why is Preventive Medicine Exempted From Ethical Constraints?', *Journal of Medical Ethics*, vol. 16, pp. 187-90.

Verbeek, A.L.M. (et al.) (1984), 'The Reduction of Breast Cancer Mortality Through Mass Screening With Mammography: first results of the Nijimegen trial', *The Lancet*, vol.1, pp. 1222-4, 2 June.

Women's National Commission (1985), *Women and the NHS*, Report of an ad hoc working group, p. 27.

World Health Organisation (1985), *World Health Statistics Annual*, WHO, Geneve.

Wright, C. (1986), 'Breast Cancer Screening: A Different Look at the Evidence', *Surgery*, vol. 100, no. 4, October.

4 The politics of homebirth: Participation versus professionalisation

K.L. Lane

The management of the delivery of pregnant women over the last hundred years has changed dramatically. The most significant development has been the continuous intervention of professionalised medical care and technology into the management and delivery of women. These changes have been described in general terms as a medicalisation of pregnancy, resulting in an increased surveillance of patients (Foucault, 1973). This medicalisation of women has major implications for the politics of health care because it has eroded the scope of women's choices over their own health. It is generally acknowledged (Oakley, 1984) that women are especially exposed to patriarchal medical systems and that women are at their most vulnerable during pregnancy. By transforming birthing into a situation of risk, medical authorities have been able to achieve almost total control over women during maternity. Yet the concept of risk is highly contestable. I argue that risk is a social, rather than a medical, category and that considerable risk is attached to the medical intervention itself. This chapter examines this issue of democracy in relation to delivery options for women in the context of a potentially radical committee report on delivery, namely the Winterton Report.

The recommendations of the Winterton Committee (1992), if they had been implemented, would have placed Britain near the forefront of maternity services within the industrialised world. The Report recommended, in general terms, the de-medicalisation of birthing. It cast doubt on the assumption that the medical model may be applied successfully to maternity care; it recognised the desirability of continuity of care by midwives, rather than GPs or obstetricians; it urged the setting up of autonomous midwifery practices undertaking total maternity care for most women; it concluded that encouraging all women to give birth in hospitals cannot be justified on the grounds of safety; it acknowledged that women are denied access to information to enable them to make truly informed choices about care; it argued that home birth or birth in small maternity units should be freely available to women; and it rejected the routine application of technology and medical intervention. Finally, the Report asserted that the hospital environment often deterred women from asserting control over their own bodies and that hospitalisation could often leave women feeling disappointed in the experience of childbirth.

The Winterton Report signified a recognition of woman-centred birthing. It amounted to a shift away from technological medicine and a move towards a more non-interventionist approach. We can call this the lay alternative or model. It recognises that pregnancy is not an illness, that the majority of women are categorised as 'low risk', and that technology should be used judiciously. Since 98 per cent of women in Britain now give birth in hospital, and because many do so on the grounds that it is only safe place to deliver, the sudden rejection of taken-for-granted assumptions represented a radical shift in public policy and a rejection of the unquestionable authority of medical personnel. It was probably for these reasons that Nicholas Winterton and the recommendations contained in the Report were refuted in the government's response. In her reply (Department of Health (DoH), *Maternity Services*, July 1992), the Secretary of State for Health underscored the DoH's continued support for medicalised birth and obstetric dominance. While the government's reply briefly alluded to the desirability of women being able to choose a low technology environment, this was overwhelmingly conceptualised as a small, medical unit. Homebirth was barely mentioned. The noticeable aspect of maternity policy is that medicalisation of birth have been profoundly successful, especially in the post-war era. This is now likely to continue in the foreseeable future.

I argue in this chapter that medicalisation has been achieved by appeal to the notion of 'risk', but 'risk' is a social, rather than a medical category. Although birthing does involve risk to life and health, the risk is associated with factors which exist socially and historically. For example, the major risks to women are medical intervention itself. However, there are also historical factors producing poor health. These historical factors include low income, poor diet, and smoking - factors which are associated with the manual social class. The argument that risk is a social, rather than a medical, category is counterposed to the implicit medical assumption that bodies are themselves inherently risky, or pathological. The medical argument locates risk within the body and consequently justifies external intervention to ameliorate the pathology. Critics of medicalised birthing have proposed that hospital is not the safest place to give birth. One critic (Tew, 1990, 1991) has produced statistical evidence to show that it is between six and twelve times safer for the majority of women to birth at home or in a small general practitioner unit (GPU) attended by a known midwife, than in a high-technological obstetric unit attended by an obstetrician. Further, even so-called 'high-risk' cases are safer at home with a midwife.

The medicalisation of birth

Foucault (1973) has argued that medical care in the newly industrialised societies of the seventeenth century shifted the role of the hospital from a place of refuge for the poor and homeless to an institution for training medical staff. It also accompanied the professionalisation of doctors, whose entry was made conditional upon the acquisition of accredited knowledge. Hospitals became places to treat the sick but, reciprocally, the sick became objects of scientific inquiry and research. In hospital, people assumed the role of patient, and patients became subject to scrutiny and surveillance by medical experts. Inevitably, this model required compliance and submission on the part of the patient so that the expert's medical knowledge could be applied.

The argument that birth has been medicalised is no longer new or surprising (see Davis and Kitzinger, 1978; Oakley, 1980, 1981, 1984, 1990; Beech, 1991; Katz-Rothman, 1982). It is less evident that medicalisation of birth has colonised the terms of the debate about birthing. To judge success or otherwise in terms of what risk attends the mother and child, is itself a medically-imposed criterion. Medical practitioners rarely consider that the mother and/or father may have alternative measures of success, or that these measures are as important as the risk of death and injury. For example, medical notes habitually exclude any evaluation of whether the mother felt satisfied with the entire series of events leading up to birth, or to what extent the mother enjoyed the experience. For medical practitioners, the 'event' has been eclipsed at around six weeks proceeding the birth. Any subsequent problems would be assessed within paediatric, gynaecological, or general health categories.

In the discussion that follows, medicalisation will be explained in terms of four major causal factors - the dominance of obstetricians and general practitioners over midwives, which constitutes a professionalised network; the concommitant acceptance of the medical-model approach to birthing (as opposed to a 'woman-centred' lay approach); the hierarchical nature of hospitalisation; and the institutionalisation of patriarchy within the medical field. Survey evidence which seriously challenge the authenticity of the medical model will be presented.

The medicalisation of birth entails a process whereby birth has been transformed from a normal, domestic event into a public medical one, that is, a situation of danger, risk and pathology. With medicalisation, the mother becomes a patient and it is supposed that she will assume the characteristics of a patient - that is, someone who is naive, passive, subordinate, and compliant. The major relationship under medicalisation has shifted from mother/baby to doctor/baby where the doctor exercises exclusive control over technology in order to achieve total control over mother and baby. By transforming birth into a situation of risk, doctors have been able to justify supervision, control and intervention over all stages of pregnancy - antenatal care, delivery and postnatal care. In this century, doctors have also been able to persuade women that unless they submit to hospitalisation and other monitoring procedures, they will expose themselves and their babies to a high risk of death and/or injury. This general climate of threat and medical repression surrounding birth continues to prevail in the majority of obstetric hospitals. It has been exercised at both a national policy and clinical/personal level. The release of the Winterton Report is the only significant inquiry in this century, at a public policy level, to question the medical-model approach to birthing and the dominance of obstetricians.

The dominance of obstetricians has occurred within the general interventions of the state in medical and social care. There are three landmarks delineating these interventions - the Boer War, the First World War and the Second World War. Mass warfare brought about enormous social change, including the increasing intervention of the state into the management of public and private life. After these great social upheavals massive social programs were instituted to alleviate such problems as housing shortages, overcrowding, poor food distribution and production and poor sanitation. As a result, the health of the population increased dramatically. Doctors were quick to make the claim that lower mortality rates of mothers and babies were wholly attributable to the hospitalisation of birthing which also occurred during this period. However, lower mortality rates were due in large part to better social conditions - improved nutrition and general standards of living (Oakely, 1984; McKeown,1979; Tew, 1990). Indeed, the reduction in mortality took place when medical services for civilians were dramatically reduced (Tew, 1990, p. 88).

The argument that hospital was safer was certainly a new proposition. In 1871, for example, Florence Nightingale had stated that home was much safer than a lying-in hospital. These hospitals had been reserved for the very poor and were commonly regarded as places of disease and infection. It is interesting to note that the nineteenth century paradigm for a healthy pregnancy advised 'rest, good food, healthy surroundings, and avoidance of excitement' (Oakley, 1984, p. 51). The latter referred to 'conjugal enjoyments'. The prevailing view emphasised social context and social relations surrounding the pregnancy as crucially affecting mortality and morbidity outcomes. This view can be diametrically contrasted to the twentieth century perspective that pathology is endemic to the individual woman, and specifically to sluggish or pathological parts of their corporeal constitutions. By the aftermath of the Boer War, however, the notion that individual mothers were negligent and needed to be managed to reduce mortality rates had become the accepted medical view. For the first time, girls were to be instructed in the art of infant feeding and management and mothers were to be educated in childrearing practices (Oakley, 1984, pp. 34-6). Mothers' ignorance of proper care was seen to be the cause of continuing high infant mortality rate which had not declined along with mortality rates generally. Infant mortality in 1900 stood at 154 per 1,000 live births, whereas the overall national mortality rate had dropped from 22.7 in 1875 to 16.9 in 1901 (Oakley, 1984, p. 37).

From 1904, working class women who experienced inadequate housing and who had little domestic help were encouraged to birth in hospital. The hospital mortality rate was still high, but hospital was considered safer for those with poor housing and for those women with obvious complications (Oakley, 1984, p. 47). Pregnancy was still seen as an essentially healthy state, but by this time antenatal care came to be regarded as a separate area of medical knowledge (Oakley,1984, p. 47).

The problem of poor housing also prompted new moves towards hospitalisation at the end of the First World War when the Local Government Board proposed the establishment of maternity homes. These were to be staffed by midwives and doctors who would attend only in emergencies. This regime belied the assumption that pregnancy and birthing were not yet regarded as pathological, or potentially pathological, states (Campbell and Macfarlane, 1987, p. 10). This was to come by the 1920s. By 1919 the new Ministry of Health established a division of Maternity and Child Welfare and, with the shift from local to national administration of health policies and the creation of more maternity homes and hospitals, birthing began a slow transferral from home to hospital. For the first time, both normal and abnormal maternity cases were regarded as appropriate for institutionalisation. It was in this era of the shift from home to hospital, that doctors also came to be regarded as appropriate managers of delivery, although midwives were not superseded until the 1950s. By the 1920s, the idea that the individual was the logical site of pathology became firmly rooted in medical discourse. Official reports considered that the high rates of maternal mortality and morbidity were attributable to the ignorance, apathy or stupidity of the mothers themselves (Oakley, 1984, p. 73). With the wide spread acceptance of the idea of individual pathology, medical concentration on mothers, by providing better antenatal services, was a logical step. Antenatal instruction was included in the medical curriculum in 1923, and in 1929 The British College of Obstetricians and Gynaecologists was founded with the intention of raising the status of antenatal care and the status of obstetricians within the medical tug-of-war over who should care for pregnant women.

The individuation of antenatal care was somewhat counteracted during the Second World War with the rise of the modern welfare state with its more holistic view of preventive medicine. During the war, for example, the introduction of free milk and school meals served to redistribute resources to low-income families. In 1941 vitamin supplements were added to blackcurrant syrup and puree to counteract shortages in butter, eggs and oranges, and from 1944 milk was fortified with Vitamin D (Oakley, 1984, p. 123). In 1942 these provisions were extended to expectant and nursing mothers and young children. By the mid-1940s, mortality rates for babies (0.36 per 1,000) and mothers (0.46 per 1,000) were the lowest on record, whilst the birth rate was the highest (Oakley, 1984, p. 127). It was on these grounds that the Royal College of Obstetricians and Gynaecologists (RCOG) recommended that hospital accommodation be provided for 70 per cent of all births on the assumption that lower mortality rates could be attributed to increased hospitalisation. Yet they did not consider, or did not wish to consider, the fact that the whole population was healthier as a result of full employment, the instigation of food subsidies, price controls, welfare foods and absence of epidemics (Oakley, 1984, p. 127).

The creation of the National Health Service (NHS) in 1948 brought about a further institutionalisation of the medical model. Intense professional conflict between GPs, specialist obstetricians situated in hospitals, and midwives attached to local health authorities providing domiciliary services was resolved by the virtual demolition of local authority responsibility for health and with it, midwifery autonomy. Thereafter, the NHS channelled pregnant women into GP surgeries and obstetric hospital units. By the late 1950s, attendance and delivery at hospital clinics exceeded local authority clinics by 2:1 (Oakely, 1984, p. 144). The incredibly low rate of maternity mortality in 1951 (0.76 per 1,000 births in England and Wales) further fuelled the unproven assertion by health authorities that hospital attendance had caused the decline. In 1959 the myth of the greater safety of hospital birth was enshrined in government policy via the Cranbrook Committee (1959) which recommended, like the RCOG, that 70 per cent of births should occur in hospitals. This trend continued well into the 1970s and 1980s. The Peel Report in 1970 urged hospital confinement for all maternity cases on grounds of safety and in 1971 the Sheldon Report extended the parameters of the medical model to include the surveillance of babies. Falling birth rates in the 1970s also led to the claim that rationalisation could be achieved by closing small GP units (GPUs) and by channelling resources towards large, intensive-care, obstetric units in hospitals. By 1980, the Social Services Committee of the House of Commons confirmed that more mothers should be delivered in large units and that home delivery and GPUs should be phased out completely. By 1991, 98 per cent of women were delivered in hospitals although, as I demonstrate later, statistical evidence could at no time support the claim that hospital was safer than home or small GPU delivery. Indeed, the case was radically the reverse.

Patriarchy and professional dominance

Inevitably the centralisation of health care, the centralisation of maternity care within large, intensive-care hospitals and the concomittant institutional dominance of obstetricians diminished the power, if not the visibility, of midwives. No longer did the midwife assume the traditional role of the advocate of the woman (that is, 'with woman') (Willis, 1983). The traditional practice that the woman held the expertise to deliver her baby while the attendant primarily encouraged and provided low-level technological and medical intervention disappeared. Hospital-based midwifery was obliged to mimic and remain subordinate to the obstetric-informed assumption that a safe birth could only be assured in retrospect. The idea that pathology can be attributed to individual bodies was naturally accompanied by the view that intervention would almost inevitably be required. Inexorably, this vision required the introduction of more numerous and more intrusive pieces of technological equipment to monitor and deliver. These practices include the routine application of scans, fetal monitoring, analgesics (including epidurals), the induction and acceleration of labour, forceps delivery, caesarian section, and non-physiological third-stage delivery. Technological birth and obstetric superiority have deskilled both women and midwives because only specialists may perform epidurals, caesarian section, induction or forceps delivery. Analytically, patriarchy and medical dominance go hand in hand. The concept can be employed to describe the historical process whereby male doctors and obstetricians have monopolised power over nurses and midwives. It can also be used to describe the doctor-patient interaction where women are rendered impotent because of their natural subordination within the gender division of labour within the household (Turner,1987, p. 102). In the final analysis, both midwives and mothers are merely women, and women are naturally subordinate to men. In this sense, argues Oakley, antenatal care and maternity care are inseparable from the treatment of women generally. The history of maternity care in her view has been a strategy for the social control of women (Oakley, 1984, p. 250).

Of considerable importance for the birthing mother is the imposition of hospital rules on the idiosyncratic nature of the birthing process. While birthing is notoriously unsuited to regimentation (if the woman is left to experience her own rhythms), the institutionalisation of birthing within the hospital system is logically geared towards uniformity of treatment and procedure. Further, as discussed above, the hospital has provided the setting for the rise of the professional dominance of obstetricians over the autonomy of midwives and mothers. The nature of the hospital as an impersonal bureaucracy, following Weber's formulation, and the notion of the hospital as incorporating a dual-structure of authority has doubly disadvantaged women and midwives. That is, one structure stems from the neutral official and 'normal' institutional procedures, and the other stems from the professional autonomy of the doctor that is core to the professional network and which is resistant to bureaucratisation (Turner, 1987, pp. 157-162).

Home or hospital and safety

In the context of this process of the institutionalisation of delivery, the Winterton Report appeared to be a sudden reversal of attitudes towards medical management. The Report recognised that 'the policy of encouraging all women to give birth in hospitals cannot be justified on grounds of safety' (p. xii). The radical note in the Report was indeed remarkable given the conceptual rigidity characterising public policy on maternity in the post-war period. Yet even this conclusion can be regarded as the more cautious end of an on-going debate within the pro-homebirth faction over exactly how much safer it is to birth at home.

The debate can be found within the respective analyses offered by Tew (1990, 1991), on the one hand, and Campbell and Macfarlane (1987), on the other. Their findings featured prominently in the collection of evidence and conclusions of the Winterton Committee. Tew, for example, has analysed both maternal and perinatal statistics in this century and has concluded that it is overwhelmingly safer for both mother and child to birth at home or in a GPU when attended by a known midwife than in an intensive-care unit in an obstetric hospital (Tew, 1990, pp. 198-298).

Taking maternal mortality statistics, Tew found that reductions in the mortality rate could be traced to the effects of social interventions associated with the war as well as pharmacological innovations, rather than to improved maternity care or medical procedures, which had remained consistent during the same period. Greater resistance to disease because of better health of mothers, and the introduction of Prontosil in 1936, which decreased death from sepsis, greatly alleviated general maternal mortality.

Table 4.1. General Maternal Mortality Rate 1930s-1950s

Year	Death Rate
1930s	0.73 - 0.86
1940	0.65
1945	0.46
1950	0.26

(Source: Tew, 1990, p. 212).

In 1937, the Chief Medical Officer of the Ministry of Health had ascertained that 40 per cent of all deaths were avoidable. Although by 1950 rates had fallen, the 'avoidable category' had not fallen at all. These were identified as - inefficiencies in the service and unsatisfactory co-operation by the mother. The statistical breakdown showed that 56 per cent in the 'avoidable category' were due to either obstetric or anaesthetist staff, 13 per cent to GPs, 23 per cent to patients and less than 2 per cent to midwives (Tew, 1990, p. 224). Further, in 1979-81, the principal causes of death - hypertensive conditions, pulmonary embolism, anaesthetic complications, and amniotic fluid embolism - were more likely to follow obstetric interventions (Tew,1990, p.

225). Tew concluded that 'the higher mortality rates in total and at specific risk levels, and the lack of association between increased hospitalisation and reduced mortality, are strong indications that obstetric interventions as a whole have not made birth safer for the mother' (Tew, 1990, p. 225).

Tew also examined infant mortality rates and was able to show that it was not only decisively safer for the majority of women (that is, low-risk women) to birth at home or in a small GPU but that, even more remarkably, the so-called high-risk cases showed a lower mortality rate at home than in an obstetric hospital. Again infant mortality made a sudden improvement after 1940, especially for post-neonatal and late neonatal cases. Between 1905-1950, these rates fell from 76.9 to 11.1 and 15.7 to 3.3 per 1,000 respectively. The early neonatal (under one week) rate was much more impervious to improvement. It fell from 24.5 in 1906 to 15.2 in 1950. By the late 1950s, the perinatal mortality rate (PNMR) seemed to recede. Rates continued to decline, but at a much slower rates. Specifically, between 1939-48 the PNMR fell by 34 per cent, but between 1949 and 1959 the rate of decline was only 8 per cent. In 1954, the rate (38.1 per 1,000 births) stood at the same level as it had in 1949 (Tew, 1990, p. 238). To ascertain the reasons for this, a national epidemiological survey was carried out in 1958. The data showed that the PNMR was highest in obstetric hospitals (50 per 1,000 births) compared with 20.3 in GPUs and 19.8 at home (Tew, 1990, p. 240). Obstetricians argued that the higher rates for hospital had occurred because the statistics were based on where delivery actually took place, and that this figure included the high mortality rate for transferred cases. Therefore, the hospital rates included high-risk cases which unfairly augmented the numbers, and unfairly diminished the numbers for home-births. It was more accurate, they argued, to base statistical analysis on the place of booking, rather than the place of delivery.

Tew has argued the reverse! It is more accurate to read the statistics from the place where care is actually received because transferred cases are those which are transferred to receive remedial treatment. The intention is to reduce the risk of mortality. If the treatment received, or the transferral itself, results in mortality (that is, it heightens the risk to an already high-risk infant, whose dubious health status cannot withstand the shock of intervention or movement) then the statistic should be allocated to the category of place of treatment, rather than the place of booking. Specifically, transferred cases should properly be designated to the hospital, because that is where the treatment was initiated. Similarly, a resulting mortality should not be attributed to home where the trauma would not have been realised (Tew, 1990, pp. 240-241). Of course, this conclusion is highly problematic for obstetricians, because it implies that it is the intervention itself, and/or the movement involved in the transfer, which is the cause of death, rather than a pathology attributed to the infant. Tew's argument rests on the premise that an already high-risk infant cannot withstand the further stress of dramatic intrusion of any kind. Death following transfers can thus be categorised under iatrogenic causes. Obstetricians have insisted, however, that PNMR rates be analysed according to booking rather than place of delivery.

When the 1958 statistics for births and perinatal rates were analysed at places of birth and at different levels of risk, it was found that it was much safer for infants to be born at home, even in the high-risk categories. It was true that a higher proportion of births occurred in hospital in all high-risk categories, but the number of high-risk cases represented only a slight increase. The slightly higher proportion of hospital births in the higher-risk categories cannot explain the fact that the mortality rates at all grades of risk, and the overall rate, were much higher for hospital than for home (Tew, 1990, pp. 242-3). The danger to the infant of hospitalised delivery was further highlighted by the fact that, for low-weight babies (which is the category accounting for the largest proportion of deaths) the rate was higher for hospital-delivery. This finding was true for two periods (1954-64 and 1967-73) in which statistics were collected. In the low-weight category, specific birthweights were analysed and showed that for babies weighing over 1500 grams the hospital rate was significantly higher. For babies weighing under 1500 grams, the place of delivery made no difference to survival (Tew, 1990, pp. 248-9).

The second national survey comprising 16,815 cases from 1970 similarly showed that the PNMR in consultant obstetric hospitals was 27.8 per 1,000 , 9.5 in general practitioner beds in obstetric hospitals, 5.4 in unattached GPUs and 4.3 at home. Because the proportion of births, but not deaths, were published in each subgroup at each place, an indirect method of standardisation was carried out. The conclusion was that 'hardly any of the hospitals' excess mortality was due to their excess of births at high risk on account of maternal age and parity' (Tew, 1990, p. 251). The same statistics were analysed to account for the combined effects of various risks. These prediction scores were called the antenatal prediction score (APS), which combined risks associated with maternal age, number of previous births, social class and known obstetric and medical risks and the labour prediction score (LPS) (the combined risk of serious complications identified during labour). The scores removed the problem of selective booking and transfers, because groups of births with the same risk score could be compared. The outcome of these calculations showed that for the APS it was much safer, even for high risk cases, to birth at home. Indeed, the rate for the low-risk group in hospital was far higher than for the high-risk group in a GPU or home - 19.3 compared with 11.0. Also only a small proportion of the excess mortality rate for hospital births could be due to the greater numbers of moderate and high risk cases due to selective bookings and early transfers (Tew, 1990, p. 254). For the LPS, the results again showed that the rate for high-risk births in a GPU or at home (14.2) was lower than for low-risk births in hospital (17.0). Further, standardisation of the figures (showing what they would have been if each place had the same proportion of births at each level of risk) indicate that very little of the hospitals' excess mortality was explicable in terms of greater numbers of births, whether transferred to hospital or actually booked to deliver there (Tew,1990, p. 255).

Campbell and Macfarlane of the National Perinatal Epidemiology Unit at Oxford have challenged the above conclusions regarding the margin of safety depicted by Tew's analyses. A review of the same statistical evidence, and other studies comparing home and hospital confinement, led them to the more minimal conclusion that 'There is no evidence to support the claim that the safest policy is for all women to give birth in hospital' (Campbell and Macfarlane, 1987, p.58). While they have ventured to suggest that there may be iatrogenic risk attached to institutional delivery for some women, they are not willing to assert this conclusively. The problem they envisaged is the variation in selection criteria which cannot be accurately measured or accounted for. They concluded, therefore, that it is not possible to assess morbidity rates according to place of birth (Campbell and Macfarlane, 1987, p. 54). Tew would assert that even if unaccountable selection biases did influence the results, the great disparity in the figures between hospital and home, particularly when the figures are standardised, could be accounted for only to a very small extent by intangible subjective factors. In her analyses, the APS and LPS incorporated all known and identified risk factors before the pregnancy and during the delivery.

For Tew, the culpable element in infant mortality was the intervention itself. Thus, the place of birth was also a proxy for the type of care received. To ascertain the difference in types of care, she analysed, in conjunction with a Dutch physician Damstra-Wijmenga, the national perinatal statistics collected in the Netherlands in 1986. Dutch statistics provided an obvious benchmark because the Netherlands remains the only developed Western country still hosting a large enough percentage of births at home under the supervision of independent midwives to provide an adequate statistical comparison. (1) The problem with UK statistics is that after 1970 almost all births occurred in hospitals. In the Netherlands by 1986, 36 per cent of all births still occurred at home. By comparing the care received by different attendants in different locations, Tew was able to show that midwifery care was a key variable in securing safety, whether or not the birth took place in hospital or at home. The mortality rate for mature babies (that is, those after 32 weeks' gestation) was almost twelve times lower if the birth occurred under midwives' care whether in hospital or at home (1.0) in contrast to the obstetricians' care in hospital (11.9) (Tew, 1991, p. 59). Qualification must be made, however, for the Dutch law states that serious conditions must be transferred to obstetric care in hospitals. Because it was not possible to ascertain what pre-delivery risk may occur to augment obstetric figures, Tew assessed the number of cases of intrauterine death, deaths due to congential malformation and preterm births occurring under midwives and obstetricians' care. She found that the stillbirth rate per 1,000 births was 11.6 for hospital obstetricians and 0.6 for all midwives. Deaths due to congenital malformation were, overall, very low in the Netherlands and the PNMR for preterm births (6.7 per cent of the total) was 85.7 for obstetricians compared with 30.0 for midwives. Thus, although obstetricians probably did deal with higher-risk cases, the differences in the PNMR at all levels of risk could not account for the disparity (a factor of twelve) in the rates accruing to obstetricians compared with midwives. Tew concluded that it was not only low-interventionist midwifery care which accounted for the greater safety of homebirth, but the setting itself which accorded to the mother the emotional security of a known and predictable environment (Tew, 1991, pp. 60-2). This argument, drawn from a number of statistical and comparative sources, reinforces the well known aphorism of French obstetrician, Michel Odent, who has professed that the greatest risk to morbidity and mortality is fear.

It is well known that the medical profession has vigorously resisted the implications of Tew's findings, which concern the iatrogenic risk to women being delivered under professional control in bureaucratic settings. It is the medical model, after all, which legitimises their control over women. Their professional interests preclude democratic choice and put women under unnecessary risk.

Consequence

Medicalisation of childbirth has seriously detracted from optimal physical outcome. Medicalisation has involved higher rates of infant mortality (Tew, 1990, 1991; Inch,

1989; Kloosterman, 1978), higher rates of intervention (Tew, 1990; Inch, 1989; WHO, 1985; Shearer, 1985; Mehl, 1978; Klein et al., 1983), and higher rates of morbidity for women and babies (Richards, 1978; Damstra-Wijmenga, 1984; Flint and Poulengeris, 1987; Alment, 1967; Klein et al., l983; Shearer, 1985,; Mehl, 1978).

Yet even the critical literature fails to mention in any detail the effects of medical interventions and morbidity outcomes on the social relations surrounding the birth and proceeding the birth. Nor does the critical literature generally appreciate the loss of power experienced by the mother, or the long-term effects such as loss of self-esteem, lack of confidence regarding her body and relationships generally, including sexual relations with her partner, impaired relations between mother and baby, and between other members of the family. With the exception of Kitzinger (1987), Tew (1990), WHO (1985) and Oakley (1981), the critical literature has failed to document the range of positive responses experienced by the few women who do manage to control the events surrounding the birth to their own satisfaction. The result is that issues such as power in the birthplace, autonomy, self-esteem and self-identity have been denied a place in birthing literature and, most visibly, in medical training. Yet it is precisely these subjective terms ('wonderful','very powerful', 'self-satisfied', 'horrid', 'terrible', 'unsupportive', 'intimidating') which women use to describe their engage-ment with childbirth and with medical personnel. Thus, to deny the language of subjectivity a place in medical discourse and to subsume all other perspectives under the language of technique and science, is at the same time to deny women a foremost position in childbirth procedures. Further, the principal role of women in childbirth is the cornerstone of women's equal participation in society generally. Democracy not only entails ownership of one's rationality, but more fundamentally, ownership of one's body.

Advances have been made within obstetric practices in hospitals as a consequence of persistent efforts by consumer-led organisations in the post-war period to humanise medical regimes. These organisations include what is now called the National Childbirth Trust, the Association for Improvements in Maternity Services, Maternity Alliance and the Active Birth Movement. The Association for Radical Midwives has also supported a pro-woman approach to birthing, because this orientation also supports their own concern at the deskilling of midwives under the medical model and hospitalisation. While obstetric practice has taken heed of a growing consumer-led movement away from the impersonalised institutional approach to birthing, these changes can only be described as cosmetic; they are only inconsistently incorporated into hospital policy. The more 'progressive' institutions may redecorate the labour room to allow flowered bedspreads, tasteful pictures and potplants, or allow fathers or chosen companions to be present at delivery. The hospital may even permit champagne in the post-delivery room and women are now spared the indignities of enemas and pubic hair shaving. However, it remains inescapable that under rational, technological management the medical model with its routinised interventions and asymmetric power relations prevail. Organised consumer response over the past thirty years (admittedly some of which has been more conciliatory than confrontative) has tried to bring about a more balanced social view of childbirth. However, pregnant women remain defined only in terms of what risk they represent to obstetric managers. Many are designated as low-risk, but they are risk-takers all the same. Thus, to be pregnant is to place oneself at risk which is the same as saying that any physiological process places one's mortality at risk. Therefore it is risky to have a heart and risky to have a liver just as it is risky for women to have a womb. All are sites of potential pathology.

Obstetricians have not only colonised women's bodies, they have colonised the terms of the debate. A successful birth, in medical terms, is one where death is avoided, that is, where woman and child remain alive after six weeks following delivery. This is an entirely technical, unnervingly narrow and passive definition of success. Why is it not equally pertinent to ask whether the woman enjoyed her birth? Why is success defined in terms of mortality? Why don't we ask whether the child was traumatised far beyond the six week period, whether the woman's relationships in wider social circles were damaged by the trauma of intervention, or whether familial dynamics were lastingly impaired? These questions are seen to be entirely irrelevant to medical ethics and this is why medical interventions occur with no thought for the damage they may cause to relations proceeding the birth. Survival is a quantitative measure of medical success, not a qualitative assessment of life. Yet it is common to hear women who delivered many years previously to recount the event in vivid emotional detail. Usually, the memory is one associated with negative emotions such as anger, resentment, fear and humiliation. Such is the commonplace negation of the validity of these long term emotional legacies that the idea of post-partum counselling remains completely extrinsic to medical practices. Of course, this negation is logical from a medical point of view, because to admit widespread long-term trauma would be to admit medical failure or at least incompetence.

Conclusion

I have argued that this century has witnessed a remarkable transition in the process of birthing. A normal physiological and cultural event has been transformed into a situation characterised by risk, danger and pathology. In short, birthing has been medicalised and there are networks and institutions which promote that medicalisation. Women are now subject to professional dominance and impersonal bureaucratisation under hospital regimes. Control over women's bodies and women's expertise have been achieved by recourse to claims about security and the essential risk entailed in all birthing procedures. Consumer-led lobby groups have been active in the post-war period to reclaim for women a more participatory role, although some of these groups have been more conciliatory than confrontative. The demand for homebirth is a confrontative strategy because it suggests that hospitalisation and attendance by obstetricians are antithetical to safe and/or pleasurable birthing. Homebirth also challenges professional dominance and networks, because women who birth at home typically seek control over all procedures and decisions. The Winterton Report has been the only document, at a public policy level, to take up the challenge against the professionalisation and bureaucratisation of birthing. Remarkably, given fifty years of entrenched conservatism in all industrialised countries, with the possible exception of the Netherlands, the Report has positively acknowledged that women desire control over their own bodies. The Report stated that women's needs were not being met. Predictably, perhaps, Winterton's recommendations were almost completely refuted by the government. In her reply, the Secretary of State for Health said that record low levels of maternal and infant mortality could be attributed to the NHS, to the 'dedication and skill of the professionals who care for our mothers and babies' and that 'advances in technology have played a significant part in this achievement' (DoH, 1992,P- 3).

In this paper, I have argued that measures of success include more than the narrow benchmark indicated by maternal and infant mortality. Participation in the decisions concerning life-chances and one's own destiny is one of the requisites of a modern democracy. Unless women participate fully in birthing, they will continue to be denied the full rights of citizenship within a modern democracy.

Footnote

1) The term 'independent' incorporates the Dutch practice of training midwives to act as autonomous professionals. This is contrasted with the British system, where midwives are trained first as nurses, and then proceed to midwifery training. The difference is that the British system effectively trains midwives to act as obstetric nurses under the auspices of the interventionist, medical model of maternity care.

Bibliography/references

Alment E.A.J., Barr A., Reid M., Reid J.J.A., (1967), 'Normal confinement: a domiciliary and hospital study', *British Medical Journal*, vol. 2.

Antonis, B. (1981), 'Mothering and Motherhood', in, Cambridge Women's Studies Group (ed), *Women in Society*, Virago, London.

Arms, S. (1975), *Immaculate Deception*, Houghton Mifflin, Boston.

Beech, B. (1991), *Who's Having Your Baby? A Health Rights Handbook for Maternity Care*, Bedford Square Press, London.

Breen, D. (1975), *The Birth of a First Child*, Tavistock, London.

Callaway H. (1978), '"The Most Essential Female Function of All" : Giving Birth', in, Ardener, S. (ed.), *Defining Females*, Croom Helm, London.

Campbell, R and Macfarlane, A. (1987), *Where to be born: The debate and the evidence*, National Perinatal Epidemiology Unit, Oxford.

Caplan, M. and Madeley, R.J. (1985), 'Home deliveries in Nottingham 1980-81', *Public Health*, vol. 99, pp. 307-13.

Cox, C.A., Fox, J.S., Zinkin, P.N., and Matthews, A.E.B., (1976),'Critical appraisal of domiciliary obstetric and neonatal practice', *British Medical Journal*, vol. 1, p. 84.

Damstra-Wijmenga, S. (1984), 'Home confinement: the positive results in Holland', *Journal of the Royal College of General Practitioners*, vol. 34, pp. 425-30.

Davis, J. and Kitzinger, S. (eds), (1978), *Place of Birth*, Oxford University Press, Oxford.

DoH (Department of Health) (1992), *Maternity Services*, HMSO, London.

Edinburgh Health Council, (1987), *User's Opinions' Survey of Lothian Maternity Services*, Edinburgh Health Council's Working Group on Maternity Services.

Fleury, P.M., (1967), *Maternity Care: Mothers' Experience of Childbirth*, Allen &

Unwin, London.

Flint, C. and Poulengeris, P. (1987), *The Know-Your-Midwife Report*, 49 Peckarmans Wood, London.

Foucault, M. (1973), *The Birth of the Clinic*, Tavistock, London.

Goldthorp, W.O. and Richman, J. (1974), 'A Case Study of the Effects of the Hospital Strike upon Domiciliary Confinement', *The Practitioner*, vol. 212, pp. 845-53.

Graham, H. (1976), 'The social image of pregnancy: pregnancy as spirit possession', *Sociological Review*, vol. 24, 291.

Haire, D. (1972),*The Cultural Warping of Childbirth*, International Childbirth Education Association, New Jersey.

House of Commons Health Committee, (1992), *Second Report, Maternity Services, Vol. 1*, HMSO, London (The Winterton Report).

Hubert, J. (1974), 'Belief and reality: social factors in pregnancy and childbirth', in, Richards, M.P.M. (ed), *The Integration of a Child into a Social World*, Cambridge University Press, Cambridge.

Inch, S. (1982), *Birthrights: A Parents' Guide to Modern Childbirth*, Green Print, London.

Ratz Rothman B. (1982), *In Labour: Women and Power in the Birthplace*, Junction Books Ltd, Great Britain.

Kitzinger, S. (1971), *Giving Birth: The Parents' Emotions in Childbirth*, Victor Gollancz, London.

Kitzinger, S. (1987), *The Experience of Childbirth*, Penguin Books, Harmondsworth.

Klein, M., Lloyd, I., Redman, C., Bull, M., Turnbull, A.C. (1983), 'A comparison of low-risk pregnant women booked for delivery in two systemsof care: shared care (consultant) and integrated general practice unit. I Obstetric procedures and newborn outcomes and II Labour and delivery management and neonatal outcome', *British Journal of Obstetrics and Gynaecology*, vol. 90, pp. 118-22 and 123-8.

Kloosterman, G.I. (1978), 'The Dutch system of home births', in, Kitzinger,S. and Davis, J. (eds), *Place of Birth*, Oxford University Press, Oxford.

Le Boyer F. (1975), *Childbirth Without Violence*, Wildwood House, London.

Lennane J. and Lennane J. (1977), *Hard Labour: a Realist's Guide to Having a Baby*, Victor Gollancz, London.

McKeown, T. (1989), *The Role of Medicine*, Basil Blackwell, Oxford.

Martin, E. (1987), *The Woman in the Body: A cultural analysis of reproduction*, Open University Press, Milton Keynes.

Mehl, L.E. (1978), 'The outcome of home delivery: research in the United States', in, Kitzinger, S. and Davis, J.A. (eds.), *The Place of Birth*, Oxford University Press, Oxford.

National Childbirth Trust (1991), *NCT Maternity Services Survey*, The National Childbirth Trust, London.

Oakley, A. (1980), *Women Confined: Towards a Sociology of Childbirth*, Martin Robertson, Oxford.

Oakley, A. (1981), *From Here to Maternity: Becoming a Mother*, Penguin, Harmondsworth.

Oakley, A. (1984), *The Captured Womb: A History of the Medical Care of Pregnant*

Women, Basil Blackwell, Oxford.

Oakley, A. (1990), 'Women as Maternity Cases', in, O'Barr, J.F., Pope, D., and Wyer, M. (eds), *Ties That Bind: Essays on Mothering and Patriarchy*, University of Chicago Press, Chicago.

O'Brien, M. (1978), 'Home and hospital confinement: a comparison of the experiences of mothers having home and hospital confinements', *Journal Royal College General Practitioners*, vol. 28, pp. 460-6.

Richards, M.P.M. (1978), 'A place of safety? An examination of the risks of hospital delivery', in, Ritzinger, S. and Davis, J. (eds), *The Place of Birth*, Oxford University Press, Oxford.

Rosengren W. (1962), 'Social status, attitudes towards pregnancy and childbearing attitudes', *Social Forces*, vol. 41.

Shaw, N.S. (1974), *Forced Labour: Maternity Care in the United States*, Pergamon Press, London.

Shearer, J.M.L. (1985), 'Five year prospective survey of risk of booking for a home birth', *British Medical Journal*, 291, pp. 1478-80.

Tew, M. (1990), *Safer Childbirth? A Critical History of Maternity Care*, Chapman and Hall, London.

Tew, M. and Damstra-Wijmenga, S.M.I. (1991), 'Safest birth attendants: recent Dutch evidence', *Midwifery*, vol. 7.

Topliss, E.P. (1970), 'Selected procedure for hospital and domiciliaryconfinements' in, McLachan, G. and Shegog, R. (eds.), *In the Beginning: Studies of Maternity Services*, Oxford University Press, Oxford.

Turner B.S. (1987), *Medical Power and Social Knowledge*, Sage, London.

Willis, E. (1983), *Medical Dominance*, George Allen and Unwin, Australia.

World Health Organisation (WHO), (1985), *Having a baby in Europe: Report on a study, Public Health in Europe 26*, World Health Organization, Copenhagen.

5 Teaching new habits: The case of AIDS

John Street

Prevention has not been the only feature of AIDS policy, but it is undoubtedly the one that has received most public attention, and arguably it is the one that is most important. For as long as there is no cure for AIDS (Acquired Immune Deficiency Syndrome) and no vaccine against it, and for as long as its spread continues to make it one of the major threats to global public health, then preventive measures generally, and public education in particular, is likely to dominate the response to the disease. But it would be wrong to attribute the prominence accorded prevention simply to the medical problems being faced. AIDS prevention policy, and especially the public education campaign, have been profoundly affected by a range of political interests and values. And it is the political process that is the concern of this chapter. (1)

In Britain, it has been the government's public education campaigns that have defined the public perception of AIDS policy. In 1986-7, British television and cinema screens showed adverts warning of the threat of AIDS and every home received a leaflet on the disease and how to avoid it. This deluge was the legacy of a watershed in British AIDS policy. In November 1986, the Thatcher government announced a major new policy initiative on AIDS. A special Cabinet Committee was to coordinate policy and there was to be a substantial increase in funding, most notably £20 million for health education campaigns. (2)

The formal purpose of British AIDS prevention policy has been to change behaviour in ways that prevent the transfer of the HIV virus, the cause of AIDS. To do this, the intention has been, first, to explain how HIV is caught, and second, to encourage practices which decrease risk of infection. The methods used for conveying these messages have extended from the high-profile media campaigns to school education packs. Their focus has ranged from sex to drug use to employment practices. Their target groups have included gays, heterosexuals, bisexuals, the young, women, ethnic groups and holiday makers.

This general goal has been served primarily by the advertising and other exercises in public education. But there have been other elements incorporated into the policy, from phone helplines to needle exchanges to the screening of blood transfusions. And importantly, within this range of options, different priorities and different degrees of commitment operate. Furthermore, there are gaps. Little has been done, for example, to stem the spread of AIDS in prison or to counter discrimination against those with AIDS.

AIDS prevention policy has, therefore, no single form, nor is it driven by a single logic. Its complex contours and lacunae are, after all, what constitute its politics. To offer a broad initial generalisation, the policy has been forged largely in the individual model, although there are the tentative gestures towards the community and systemic models. The focus has been on 'at risk' individuals and groups; it has had little to say about the causes of 'risky behaviour' or the wider context of social action.

It might be tempting to explain the preference of the individual model by reference to the nature of the disease and its transmission, but such an account immediately meets the problem that other governments faced by the same disease have adopted quite different preventive policies (Kirp and Bayer, 1992). Rather, an explanation of the character of British AIDS prevention policy must focus on the character of the policy community and policy networks that have shaped the response to AIDS. Such an examination reveals three key factors: (i) the dominance of the medical profession and the marginalisation of the voluntary sector; (ii) the impact of (party) political values on policy; and (iii) the influence of institutional practices and precedents on AIDS prevention. To appreciate how these factors played their part, we need first to provide a brief sketch of the way AIDS emerged in Britain.

HIV and AIDS in Britain

The first recorded death from AIDS in Britain was in 1982. Subsequently, in the period to December 1990, 4098 people contracted AIDS, of which nearly 50 per cent had died by the end of the decade. This raw data tells us little and needs to be subdivided. The Department of Health (DoH) statistics distinguish between people with AIDS by bracketing them according to the route by which HIV was thought to be contracted (see Table 5.1).

The distribution of AIDS provides only a partial explanation of the way in which the prevention policy has operated. There is no neat correlation between who has AIDS and the focusing of the advertising campaigns. While the distribution helps to explain the advertisements aimed at the tourist, it does not account for the focus on the heterosexual population in general or the lack of attention on the drug user. Perhaps more important, though, is the set of judgements incorporated into the policy in the way the statistics themselves are presented. The distribution of the disease is measured by reference to *social/medical categories* rather than *sexual or other practices*. This is

Table 5.1. People With AIDS (December 1990)

Category	
Homo/Bisexual	3234
IVDA (intravenous drug abuse)	161
Homo/Bi + IVDA	61
Haemophiliac	228
Blood Recipient	
abroad	37
UK	30
Heterosexual contact	
Partner with above risk factor	34
Others Abroad	208
No evidence of exposure abroad	26
Child of at risk/infected parent	36
Other	43
Total	4098

(Source: Department of Health)

indicative of the way AIDS prevention policy is thought about, as something that has to be targeted at recognisable groupings. At the same time, looking at the subtext of the statistics does not account for the language of the advertising or for the range of elements and strategies contained within prevention policy generally. In the first instance, understanding and explaining the preventive response to AIDS means going beyond the official statistics, and to examining how the 'problem' was perceived.

The emergence of an AIDS policy

How these figures take on political salience depends on the political processes by which they were converted into the 'problem' of AIDS. There were two elements to this process. There was the role played by the media and the role played by the official policy machine in the DoH and the National Health Service (NHS).

The media and AIDS

The first news of AIDS was carried in the specialist media aimed at the Gay and the medical communities. Within the Gay press, news of what was happening in San Francisco received considerable coverage in the early 1980s. Journals like *The Lancet* and the *British Medical Journal* reported the emergence of a new disease. AIDS received little attention from either the mass circulation tabloids or from the 'serious' broadsheet press. The *Mail on Sunday* devoted a front-page story to the heterosexual spread of AIDS in 1983, but this did not, however, inspire any further coverage.

The populist interest in AIDS arrived later. The tabloid papers began to feature AIDS in 1985, and then gave it their most lurid coverage. From February to March, according to one observer (Naylor, 1985, p. 5), 'hardly a day would pass without it receiving national press coverage'. Headlines and stories made much of the gay connection, and played upon the homophobia that was part of the papers' staple diet. There were frequent references to the 'gay plague', 'gay menace' and 'gay killer'. Stories of the spread of AIDS referred to the 'dark corners' and 'twilight world' of homosexuals. The event that focused these attitudes was the death of a prison chaplain, Gregory Richards. Zoe Schramm-Evans (1990, p. 4) argues that this death was 'one of the most significant domestic factors' affecting 'government policy in the early years'.

Television often takes its political agenda from the press, but in the case of AIDS its coverage seems to have run independently. Certainly, its tone and focus were different. While the press fuelled public fears of AIDS, television focused more on the public policy. Although both media played their part in creating pressure for government to act, it is worth noting that AIDS received 'unprecedented coverage' on TV in the two months before the November 1986 watershed (Garland, 1987, pp. 50-2). And this coverage, unlike much that appeared in the press, addressed the question of what the government ought to do.

The importance of the media (and TV in particular) lay not just in the way it publicised the problem, but also in the way it became part of the solution. Not only was television an agent of government public health policy, it also became an influence upon it. The medium affected the message. A distinct notion of the 'public' came into play, the 'public' of public service broadcasting. Alcorn (1989) writes: 'In the UK, broadcasting was expected to respond at the point when the virus threatened to "leak" into "the general population"'. Public service broadcasting took a particular view of the public; it was heterosexual. Meanwhile, the press continued to represent the fear of homosexuality. Together the two media played a vital part in setting the agenda for the government's response to AIDS. They helped to prepare the ground for the major political intervention in AIDS policy that occurred in 1986. But such shifts cannot be explained without reference to the evolution of departmental policy.

Health policy and AIDS

Before the 1986 watershed, AIDS policy was essentially treatment policy, although some limited attempts were made at prevention through education. Relatively little of this policy was made at the centre, and detailed policy strategies emerged mainly at regional, district, and sometimes even hospital ward level. In England, the main responsibility for policy development fell to the North West Thames regional health authority and the two main district health authorities within the region, Riverside and Parkside. These were the authorities that looked after 50 per cent of people with AIDS in England.

St Mary's Hospital in Parkside houses the largest genito-urinary unit in Europe and since 1982 had been developing its services for AIDS patients. Parkside created an AIDS strategy, quite independently of the DoH. In doing so, it established a clear divide between prevention policy on the one hand and diagnosis, treatment and support policies on the other. The prevention policy emphasised the need for, first, accurate monitoring and surveillance; this was to provide a basis for community and work-place initiatives intended to raise levels of awareness and to enable people to adopt behaviour that minimised the risk of infection. In short, it attempted to introduce a community model of prevention. There were limits, however, to the Health Authorities' ability to deliver on this strategy. Without any major government commitment, funding had to come from existing budgets which were already under considerable strain. But even with the resources, it is unlikely that the community prevention strategy would have flourished. It needed cooperation with other agencies, and such a network was not adequately developed and was a constant problem of health authority practice. Furthermore, it required a commitment to prevention, and again this was not an established part of the health authorities' remit; instead, it was given low status and little attention (Beardshaw, 1989).

These problems were exacerbated by the fact that AIDS was bracketed with the treatment of sexually transmitted diseases (STDs) generally (Weeks, 1981). The low status accorded this branch of medicine hampered the redistribution of funds. It is also worth noting that, because AIDS was linked to the treatment of STDs, similar rules applied in the attempt to limit its spread. Instead of the more aggressive contact-tracing schemes developed in the USA and elsewhere (Kirp and Bayer, 1992; Bayer, 1989), the British system preserved the emphasis on anonymity and voluntarism in contact-tracing, themselves the legacy of STD policy generally.

Another important institution in the evolution of AIDS prevention policy was the Health Education Council (HEC). From relatively early in the epidemic, the HEC produced leaflets and packs on AIDS. The HEC was hampered, however, by the limits to its resources. And what impact it did have helped to reinforce the individualist model of prevention policy.

Finally, before any major political commitment, the DoH (then still joined to the Department of Social Security) was slowly developing its own response to AIDS. Relying heavily on the initiative of the Chief Medical Officer, Sir Donald Acheson, and a series of advisory committees, staffed largely by clinicians working with AIDS, the Department began to formulate strategies for treatment, prevention and research.

So prior to late 1986, within the health policy arena, there were agencies and interests organising around AIDS, and creating the basic structure of an AIDS policy and representing pressure for a particular kind of preventive response. Outside this arena was the growing public attention on AIDS. The two were combined in the November 1986 watershed. It was then that AIDS policy took on a high profile and became the beneficiary of far greater resources, particularly for prevention. This was given institutional recognition when the HEC was replaced by the more powerful Health Education Authority, which then set up a special AIDS unit. One obvious result of all this was that prevention policy became increasingly subject to political pressure.

Prevention policy and AIDS

While public perception of prevention policy has conflated it with education policy, it does not follow, as I have suggested, that this is all that prevention policy does or can involve.   To understand the politics of the policy is to explore the priorities, values and interests organised into prevention - and to see what is organised out.   What follows does not pretend to be a comprehensive review, but tries instead to show how policies and prevention have interacted.   There are three elements to the prevention policy that I want to focus upon.   The first, and most obvious, aspect is the education programme that has operated since the political watershed of 1986.   The second is the policy on condom distribution and needle exchanges.   The third looks at the less well-defined area of background attitudes to AIDS, in particular discrimination against people with HIV and AIDS.   Each one maps roughly onto the three models of prevention policy - individual, community, systemic - with which this book deals.

Public education

The programme of public education has received the most attention since it was perceived by policy makers as the only way in which the spread of HIV infection could be stemmed.   It is also the most visible aspect of AIDS policy and it carries, therefore, the greatest short-term political costs and benefits.   Its functional and political roles are not easily separated.   On the one hand it can be seen to be the only realistic response.   The minister who presided over the 1986 watershed, Norman Fowler, remarked that 'public education is the only vaccine we have' (*The Guardian*, 17 November, 1986).   At the same time, public education has the political advantage of being highly visible.   Ministers can point proudly at the public evidence of their endeavours.

Apart from the priority attached to public education, there was the matter of what message it should carry.   The DoH wanted to avoid preaching to its audience or shocking them.   The Department sought 'a way of telling people what the risks are and what they should do without shocking them so much that they switch off entirely' (*The Guardian*, 17 November, 1986).   Equally, it was recognised that 'we frankly don't have time to rely on changing the moral climate' (*The Guardian*, 22 November, 1986).   While this has remained the DoH's strategy, it has had its critics from within the government itself (including the Prime Minister).   Other departments have been less sympathetic to the non-moralistic approach.   The Department of Education and Science demanded the pulping of a schools training pack on AIDS, because the pack lacked a suitably strong moral message about sex within marriage and about the 'immorality' (and illegality for those under 21) of homosexuality (*The Observer*, 19 June, 1988).

As the main agent of the Health department's will, the Health Education Authority (HEA) has also avoided preaching and instead aimed 'to create and sustain an

Table 5.2. Publicity Campaigns

Date	Audience/location	Theme
March 1986	National press	Information
Dec 86 - Feb 87	TV, Press, Posters, Leaflets to all homes	Don't die of ignorance
Feb 88	TV, youth magazines (men and women)	You know the risks; the decision is yours
Summer 88	Posters in airports ports, stations etc	Holidays
Dec 88 - March 89	National press	You're as safe as you want to be
March 89	Gay press, listings magazines	Men who have sex with men
April 89 - June 89	Young women's mags, young women ethnic press	Young women
Summer 89	Posters at airports etc Radio, ads in inflight magazines	Holidays
Dec 1 1989	Ads in national daily, Sundays, and ethnic press	World AIDS Day
Dec '89 March 90	Ads in youth press (men women), Radio	Young people
Feb - March 90	TV, National press	Experts on HIV & AIDS

(Source: HEA, *Strategic Plan 1990-1995*)

informed climate of opinion around HIV and AIDS' (HEA, 1989). This has meant telling people how AIDS is transmitted, and how to prevent transmission (primarily through safe sex, although there is occasional reference to monogamy). These messages have been subject to close political scrutiny. Right-wing critics have demanded more explicit moral messages; while left critics of the HEA claim that it has tended to play on an implicit puritan moralism, relying too much on fear ('behind every beautiful person there is a potential carrier of HIV') to get its lesson across (*Times Higher*, 3 July, 1992, p. 18).

The HEA itself claims that its campaigns owe more to the evidence of market research than to any attempt to adopt any particular line. Its strategy is, it claims, to reach those groups who are not changing their behaviour; the message is, therefore, just a function of its target. Certainly the phases into which the campaign has been divided accord with this general strategy (see Table 5.2). While the first two campaigns, run in 1986, were largely directed at the general population, some of the subsequent ones have been more precisely focused: on the young and on intravenous drug users. Almost all the campaigns are directed at heterosexuals. The target groups, in this sense, reflect the political focus of AIDS policy. But it also reflects the fact that, through the initiative of voluntary groups like the Terrence Higgins Trust, there had already been extensive publicity directed at gay groups (Wiseman and Bodell, 1990).

The first national campaigns, directed at 'the public', were designed to increase awareness of AIDS first and then to change behaviour. But it is noticeable that the approach has been one of simply conveying information, adopting the 'hypodermic model' of communication: information is simply injected into the public, with little attention being paid to how that information is received or interpreted.

One of the early leaflets began with an injunction to 'Please read this carefully' and was signed by the government's Chief Medical Officers. It went on to explain what AIDS is, how it is spread, and how it can be avoided: 'Using a sheath can help reduce the risk of catching AIDS. So can cutting out casual relationships'. The only illustration was a picture of an AIDS leaflet.

Later material was more direct, and involved the circulation of leaflets to every home in the country, poster and billboard advertising, and TV and radio slots. It cost more than £10 million. Its intention was to encourage safer sex, which was defined as 'sticking to one partner' and/or 'use a condom'. For all this, its approach to education remained a one-dimensional exercise in public information.

This was despite a new-found willingness to make novel use of television and radio. Public service announcements may have long been a feature of British broadcasting, warning of dangers on the roads or in the home. The Thatcher government transformed this tradition. The Department of Trade and Industry employed high profile contemporary advertising techniques to promote its policies, just as other departments of state had employed advertisers to sell shares in the government's privatisation programme. The advertisements themselves were shown in January 1987, and though they were stylishly designed, they remained rather coy affairs. They served only to notify the public of the leaflet that was being sent to every home. The national AIDS helpline, together with the leaflet, was to provide the detailed public health information. The message was 'don't die of ignorance'. The government's use of advertising for its AIDS campaign was, therefore, part of its established, if evolving, practice.

What was different about AIDS, though, was that the government took an interest in the general coverage given to AIDS. The government, for example, encouraged broadcasters to lift the ban on advertising condoms. There were meetings between the Chief Medical Officer (CMO), civil servants, and senior television executives which led to the idea of a media 'AIDS Week' (Alcorn, 1990). The health education campaign thereby linked the official government strategy to the ethos of public broadcasting, with its commitments to balance and moderation.

While the informational approach has met with some success, it has not been a triumph of preventive policy making. Although the advertising campaigns have varied in their impact, the general pattern of results have indicated that people have increased in awareness of AIDS but done little to change their behaviour (Campbell and Waters, 1987; Beck et al., 1987; Kapila and Wellings, 1989). Information does not link directly to action. A poll of 18-24 year olds conducted in March 1987 revealed that while 15 per cent of respondents said that they had given up casual sex and 36 per cent said they favoured monogamy, only 2 per cent said that they used condoms. The campaign seemed not to have altered the view that AIDS was something that people caught through their own actions (DHSS, 1987). The campaign also caused people to seek tests for HIV, but again those doing so were not in the primary target group. Of people asking to be tested, the figure rose by 191 per cent among homo-/bi-sexuals, by 138 per cent among drug users, and 352 per cent among those with no known risk factor (*The Lancet*, 1987, p. 1429). As one team of researchers (Nutbeam et al., 1989) concluded, the public had been 'informed but not yet adequately educated'. It was only among gays that behaviour had changed significantly. Young heterosexuals were the most resistant to influence. There was some evidence, too, that wider social attitudes had been little affected. Prejudice against homosexuality remained as did the view that people with AIDS only had themselves to blame. The problem faced by the campaigns was neatly described by one advertising executive who observed: 'We are talking about changing a way of life. There is no point buying one page in a paper to discourage permissiveness when the other 24 promote it' (*Media Week*, 21 November, 1986). Clearly, this is not the only issue, but it is evident that the dominant form of health education has real limits based on the general theory of education deployed. The problem of theory has to be combined with the practice of politics. One particular campaign neatly illustrates this point.

In early 1990, a series of advertisements was run on prime-time TV. They had the same format: a single talking head. The talking heads were all experts in the AIDS field: Sir Donald Acheson, Professor Michael Adler, Dr. Anthony Pinching, Dr. Anne Johnson, Dr. Raymond Maw and others. Each uttered a simple statement about HIV and AIDS.

Why was this low key approach adopted? Partly it reflected a changing perception of the problem of AIDS, from that of an immediate crisis to that of a long-term policy. But there were more direct, political causes for the change of tone. There had been renewed media interest in AIDS. This time it sought to detract from the panic which had been created earlier, particularly about the heterosexual spread. *The Sunday Times* serialised the book by Michael Fumento (1990) which had cast doubt on the idea of 'heterosexual AIDS'; the same theme was taken up by various people in the letter columns of the 'serious' press; and a television documentary gave publicity to Professor Duesberg's claim that HIV was not the cause of AIDS. This new interest in the disease coincided with reports of the scrapping of the HEA's AIDS unit (HEA, 1990). It also coincided with a decline in the political fortunes of the Conservative government, as it trailed behind Labour in the opinion polls. This made the government politically sensitive to anything that might detract further from its popularity, a popularity that it had chosen to build around the family and morality.

It was in this political climate that the HEA devised the 'experts' campaign. It was designed both to maintain the credibility of the HEA and its message, conveying the necessary information in an unsensational fashion. The campaign, in short, was informed as much by the politics of the day as by the spread of the disease and the established practice of health education.

One final factor worth identifying in the construction of education policy is that of the internal institutional machine and its politics. In the mid-1980s, the CMO created the Health Education Advisory Group (HEAG) to advise on prevention policy. Although the HEAG's suggestions were sometimes overlooked, even before the 1986 watershed, its work was considered valuable by at least one member:

> Despite the fact that the *advisory* status of the Group was regularly stressed by the secretariat, and a high proportion of our unanimous suggestions were ignored or over-ruled in the subsequent (first) newspaper campaign, it provided a valuable and unique forum for discussion of these issues. It has been the most stimulating and productive of all the many groups of which I have been a member (SSSC, 1987, vol. ii, p. 35).

The HEAG undoubtedly made an impact in the early days of AIDS public education. The DoH was uncertain about how to proceed. The HEAG persuaded the CMO to focus on condom use. The Secretariat obliged by furnishing the Group with extensive documentation on condom promotion campaigns throughout the world (including Australia's 'rubber dubber' campaign). The HEAG also managed to cajole the Department into making its campaigns more explicit.

The HEAG, however, eventually fell into disuse. There were a variety of reasons for this. The HEAG's influence was, it seems, inversely proportional to the political interest taken in their work. As political responsibility for public education increased, so expertise became more selectively chosen, and groups like the Terrence Higgins Trust were pushed to one side. While the HEAG had extensive voluntary sector representation, its successor, Coordination of AIDS Public Education (CAPE), employed only established health service agencies and representatives of government departments.

It was not just politics, though, that limited the effect of the HEAG's advice. The character of that advice also mattered. The HEAG was not offering hard science, instead its advice was grounded in psychology and the study of social behaviour. This was a type of knowledge which tended to be viewed as 'common sense', despite evidence to the contrary. Reflecting upon his experience on the HEAG, the sociologist Tony Coxon remarked:

> The feeling I have, particularly, was that there was a very strong mix of concern and expertise which, in the event, was not actually used and that whilst in particular medical skills were being called upon and used and respected, other sorts of non-medical skills were being ignored (SSSC, 1987, vol. ii, p.35).

Whatever its weaknesses, the education campaign was a key component of the preventive strategy. It is worth reflecting, therefore, upon the factors that shaped it. First, there were the statistics and language which helped to define 'the problem' of AIDS. These tended together to emphasise risk groups rather than risky practices and to direct attention towards a heterosexual 'public'. Secondly, there was the way in which 'education' was represented as 'information' to be injected into that public. This was a legacy of government information provision generally. Thirdly, there were the political judgements which were made about how explicit that information should be and in what context it should be presented. And finally, there were institutional mechanisms - most obviously, the HEAG - which served to select and shape the knowledge base of the education campaign.

Needles and condoms

The Thatcher government did introduce a number of direct measures to stem the spread of AIDS. The earliest and most important of these was the decision taken in 1985 to ensure that donated blood was tested for HIV. But for the most part it remained cautious of interventions of this kind. This reluctance is most obvious in the case of its policy (or lack of policy) on condoms and needle exchanges. Condoms are one of the key defences against the sexual transmission of HIV, just as clean needles are vital to cutting down the spread among drug users. A further insight into the politics of prevention can, therefore, be gained by asking why the government has been reluctant to push condom use and needle exchanges?

While the Labour opposition advocated the free distribution of condoms, the government resisted this advice. Individual hospitals and family planning clinics distribute condoms, but doctors cannot prescribe them, although they can prescribe all other forms of contraception. This policy is a legacy of 1975 when free contraception was introduced. It was thought that condom users rarely needed medical advice and so it would be inappropriate for doctors to deal with them. Doctors failed in their campaign to change the status quo (*The Independent*, 23 July, 1990). The government also took no steps to monitor the production of condoms or to insist on new standards of safety. This has been left to the market. There has been little government encouragement to eroticise (or destigmatise) the condom. This too has been left to retailers, manufacturers and their advertisers, and voluntary bodies. Although the HEA has tried to add a note of sensuality into some of its adverts (which have otherwise tended to play on fear), the voluntary sector has been much better at presenting safe sex as erotic.

The only explicit government decision has been *not* to distribute condoms in prisons, on the grounds that this would only encourage dangerous sexual practices, which are, in any case, illegal in prison. While this constitutes a formal reason for inaction, it is hard to resist the conclusion that simple electoral calculations are also involved. The party of the family and of law and order did not wish to be associated with homosexuality in prisons.

A similar lack of action characterised the government's policy on the provision of free needles and needle exchanges. Although the CMO and the Advisory Council on the Misuse of Drugs (ACMD) had advocated a national needle exchange scheme, the government has been reluctant to follow this advice, beyond a few pilot initiatives and some encouraging noises. With the pilot schemes, pharmacists were invited to support the policy through the sale of syringes, but the basic implementation was left to local authorities. As a result, the policy took very different forms. Where there was a fierce local anti-drugs policy (as in Edinburgh) and little desire to promote needle exchanges, the spread of HIV continued to increase; where a more relaxed drug policy operated (as in Liverpool and Glasgow), the incidence of HIV was lower. Two years later, the scheme remained at the experimental stage, and ministers were voicing concern over both its effectiveness and its potential political costs. Rather than introduce a national policy, the preference was to let it remain a matter for local initiative (DoH, *Press Briefing*, 1988, 88/102). Eventually, though, the status quo was overturned.

In 1988, with the publication of a powerfully worded report from the government's own Advisory Council (ACMD), a move to a national policy was made. The government was caught in an awkward dilemma: it was committed to countering the spread of AIDS, but it was determined to stamp out drugs. This dilemma was institutionalised in the policy network. In one corner was the Home Office whose goal was the elimination of hard drugs in Britain through the use of tough law enforcement. Meanwhile, over at the DoH concern was less with preventing drug use than with hindering the spread of HIV through shared needles. Although the Home Office's campaign would, if successful, have ended worries about one aspect of the transmission of HIV, there was no guarantee of that success. The DoH strategy accepted the fact of drug use and sought to work within it. The DoH accepted, in other words, the dictum that 'HIV is a greater threat to public and individual health than drug misuse'(ACMD, 1988). The same dilemma is, of course, reproduced in prisons, but here the authority and responsibility rests almost exclusively with a single arbiter, the Home Office.

The policy on needles in prisons echoed that on condoms. Needle exchanges were ruled out by the Home Office. It argued that the incidence of intravenous drug use was small and that distributing free needles would, in fact, exacerbate the problem (DoH, 1989). It is, actually, very hard to know what the exact figures are. The incidence of HIV in prison is low - in January 1989, there were fifty men and seven women who were HIV positive in prison, but again there has been no systematic testing to identify the full extent of the problem. Meanwhile, unofficial reports suggest that the sharing of needles is quite common.

Where there was no decisive authority within the policy network, preventive policy was determined by a number of factors. One element was the report on *AIDS and Drug Misuse* (1988), produced by the ACMD and commissioned by the DoH. The committee placed HIV over drugs in its priorities, and therefore recommended that more effort be put into preventing the sharing of needles and into informing users about how to minimise the risk of infection. This meant a break with the individualist model of prevention, and entailed a move towards the community approach. The Report said:

> a change in professional and public attitudes to drug misuse is
> necessary as attitudes and policies which lead to drug misusers
> remaining hidden will impair the effectiveness of measures to
> combat the spread of HIV (ACMD, 1988, para. 2.3).

Pharmacists, GPs and others were all to be involved. These recommendations not only won the support of the CMO, they also received considerable public attention. (Many such reports, including those produced by the ACMD, had disappeared without trace or received no public notice. Indeed, the ACMD traditionally functions quietly.) In this case though, the chair of the responsible working group, Ruth Runciman, decided that a more public strategy was necessary if the government was to be persuaded to act. She made sure the press and parliament was fully briefed.

Even with the considerable publicity, the Minister at the Department, John Moore, was reluctant to move. He worried about seeming to condone or accept the use of hard drugs. There was a three month delay before he decided to publish the Advisory Council's report in March 1988. When the report was eventually made available, the government gave it a grudging endorsement, but avoided accepting its main message about prevention and risk management. While needle sharing 'presents a grave threat', argued the government:

> it is self-evident that if people do not start using drugs in the first place then they do not put themselves at risk of infection through this route. We remain therefore determined to prevent the misuse of drugs, both through tough law enforcement measures to reduce the supply of illicit drugs, and through effective education and information to make it less likely that young people will be tempted to try them (DHSS *Circular*, HC(88)26).

A similar attitude was expressed towards needle exchanges: 'Ministers believe that there is as yet insufficient evidence about the benefits or otherwise of syringe-exchange schemes to recommend expansion of schemes' (DHSS *Circular*, HC(88)26).

It was not until Moore was replaced at the Department by David Mellor (who as a Home Office Minister had some drugs expertise but who was not totally imbued with that department's ethos) that decisive action was taken. For the first time there was an official policy on drugs and AIDS which went beyond the existing *ad hoc* needle exchange scheme. In September 1988, the Department made £3 million available to Health Authorities to prevent the spread of HIV among drug users. 'Drug misusers', said David Mellor, 'must be encouraged to come forward for help' (DoH, *Press Release*, 27 August, 1988). Health Authorities were required to expand their services and support for, and links with, drug users. The story of needle exchanges, if not of condom supply, reveals again the mixture of institutional and individual factors which combine to shape prevention policy. Two factors appear to be decisive. The first concerns the balance of power (or responsibility) within the policy community. Where the DoH and the Home Office both had claims on the policy arena, prevention policy emerged as an awkward compromise of their different ambitions. The second involves the opportunity for decisive new ideas to emerge and to acquire authority. Without the catalytic role of the ACMD, it is unlikely that the needle exchange scheme would have survived at all, and prevention policy would have remained within the individualist model.

Attitudes to AIDS

While the Advisory Council on the Misuse of Drugs could do something to push the government towards a community model of prevention, little chance existed for an systemic approach to emerge. The government has not been oblivious, though, to such a strategy, but at the same time it has not offered a great deal of support for it. The formal intention has been to prevent AIDS becoming an object of fear, stigma and prejudice. (And it is evident that such a goal must link to a general concern with prevention). But if the measure of the government's commitment was an attempt to outlaw discrimination, then it has scored poorly. It has, for the most part, confined itself to well-intentioned injunctions and a reliance on existing legislation, which in a country with no Bill of Rights provides little protection (Orr, 1989).

The government has done nothing beyond issuing guidelines for those who work with HIV-positive people. No laws have been introduced to prevent discrimination against those who are HIV positive, although the Department of Employment introduced a pamphlet on *AIDS and employment* which indicated that the dismissal of anyone because they were HIV positive would be unfair under the terms of the existing legislation.

The government has done nothing to respond to complaints from the Terrence Higgins Trust and others about insurance companies who deny cover to people who are (or are suspected of being) HIV positive. The insurers do not deny the charge. They see it as their right to determine whom they cover. The chairman of the Life Insurance Council, the industry's regulatory body, told the House of Commons Select Committee: 'We are not turning people down just because they are homosexual but there is usually a medical related factor that comes in' (SSSC, 1987, vol. ii, p. 261). No one, he said, was refused insurance simply because they had had a test for HIV. But the rider was added that the Association of British Insurers, the insurers' trade representative, could not enforce an industry-wide policy on this issue, and that companies were at liberty to impose 'their own particular underwriting philosophy and standards. We are not in a position to say to a member that he has refused a case incorrectly' (SSSC, 1987, vol. ii, p. 262). The insurers therefore claim, on the one hand, that they are not making judgements on the basis of sexuality but on grounds of risk; and on the other, there is no formally imposed criteria for granting or refusing cover. The result is, of course, discrimination against people with HIV.

Despite the protests, the government has been unwilling to intervene in the activities of the insurance industry (a stance that is not exclusive to this policy area). In both their 1987 and 1989 reports, the Social Services Select Committee criticised the insurance industry and called upon the government to outlaw the AIDS-related questions. The government's only concession was to agree to meet the industry representatives to discuss the policy. This was, it seems, a mere gesture, because the government was convinced of 'the need of the insurance industry to find out relevant information before providing life insurance' (SSSC, 1989, para. 19). The reluctance to mount a systemic prevention policy owes much to the dominant view about the limits to government involvement, at least rhetorically. A more complete account, though, depends upon recognising the balance of power and interests organised around insurance policy.

Analysing AIDS prevention policy

A number of lessons can be drawn from this account of AIDS prevention policy. Just as my account has been selective, so too are my conclusions. My concern is with the way in which political processes have impinged upon policy. This impact has been measured in three areas of AIDS prevention policy - education, needle exchanges and condom supply, and discrimination. These three fit roughly into the three categories of prevention policy: individual, community, systemic. The three categories also demarcate the general priorities that have shaped government policy. The greatest emphasis has been placed upon education, and the least upon discrimination. This pattern owes something to the way the problem of AIDS has been defined (as one of individual behaviour), but it is also a consequence of the political mechanisms that have processed and shaped such perceptions. It is these to which I want to draw attention here.

There are three particular types of political impact to be discerned. The first concerns the management of the political interests around AIDS; the second focuses on the way political ideology and political actors have shaped policy; and the third looks at the policy process itself and at how its operating procedures have shaped the government's response.

1) The range of interests included in the policy community has been narrow. The consultative system has been dominated for the most part by medical-clinical expertise. This partiality is best demonstrated by the treatment of the Terrence Higgins Trust (THT). They have been kept on the fringes of policy making. Despite the expertise they developed in AIDS and in education policy, it has been little used, except by the HEA and the DoH in the early days. Their function has been confined to that of a conduit for government policy. Norman Fowler, the Minister who presided over the 1986 watershed, had few dealings with the Trust and rarely spoke of it in his public pronouncements, while one of his successors, David Mellor, visited the Trust's headquarters and was willing to acknowledge its importance to the government's overall strategy. Nonetheless, the THT's role was clearly circumscribed by government policy. Mellor used the THT 'to update and deepen my awareness of AIDS' (HC Debate, col. 100, 13 January 1989). They were part of the government's plan, according to Mellor, 'to have good links with key groups in the community' (SSSC, 1989, p. 12).

2) Prevention policy has been shaped by party political ideology. The government's reluctance to act over discrimination fitted with its general concern to limit the scope of government intervention, at least where it relates to industry. The Thatcher government was ill-disposed to intervention in the market. Equally, Mrs. Thatcher, the embodiment of that ideology, had an impact on AIDS policy but this was not always to be measured in direct intervention. Her views caused some modification to the language of the advertising campaigns and the cancellation of the National Survey of Sexual Behaviour. Hugo Young (1990, p. 548) described the circumstances of the latter decision:

The Prime Minister's veto on public money appeared to derive

from an instinctive distaste for invasion of heterosexual privacy
- although homosexuals were fair game.   Her decision was
never explicitly defended.   It simply happened, without a public
rationale and without the relevant minister, in possession of the
scientific facts, feeling able to challenge it.

The decision was not, however, simply based on a whim.   At one level, it was
consistent with her vision of normality and decency (which she saw herself as
personifying) and which required the maintenance of a particular reading of
puritanism.   It would be wrong, however, to see her as exercising a constant scrutiny
of AIDS policy.

She made few public comments on AIDS and did not take part in any of the
parliamentary discussions of AIDS (although this was entirely consistent with her
attitude to parliament generally).   Nor did she chair the Cabinet committee.   It is
apparent, though, that many policy decisions were taken in anticipation of her views.
Furthermore, the context in which AIDS policy was expected to operate was framed
by policies closely associated with her - reforms of local government (especially
Clause 28 of the Local Government Act) and cutbacks in public expenditure.

3) Standard operating procedures and the departmental ethos have played an important
role in shaping the final form of AIDS prevention policy. The contrasting behaviour
and reaction to AIDS of the DoH and the Home Office eloquently illustrate the impact
of department interests on policy.   An equivalent contrast could be made between
AIDS policy in Scotland and in England. The different institutional structure of
Scotland, and the fact that prison and health policy fall to the same department of
state, has made possible a more coherent policy on HIV in prisons.

Less easily detectable, but no less important, has been the way the enclosed, elite
administrative structure has limited the ideas and interests incorporated into preventive
policy. The health message has been delivered from on high, and has been couched in
the language of a threat to specific groups.   Paternal protectionism has been the
dominant code. And arguably, it has been less effective for this. It is hard not to notice
that the one group of people to have made most change to their behaviour are
homosexuals, the one group to whom the government has paid least attention (at least
in connection with AIDS) and who have been reached by quite different channels.

Footnotes

1) Much of the material used in this chapter is drawn from research financed by the
University of California at Berkeley and conducted in collaboration with Professor
Albert Weale at the University of East Anglia.

2) For a more detailed history of AIDS policy, see Berridge and Strong, 1990, Klein
and Day, 1990, Street and Weale, 1992.

Bibliography/references

ACMD (Advisory Council on the Misuse of Drugs) (1988), *AIDS and Drug Misuse*, vol. 1, HMSO, London.

Alcorn, K. (1989), 'AIDS in the Public Sphere', in, Carter E. and Watney, S. (eds), *Taking Liberties: AIDS and Cultural Politics*, Serpent's Tail, London, pp. 193-212.

Bayer, R. (1989), *Private Acts, Social Consequences*, Free Press, New York.

Beardshaw, V. (1989), 'Blunted Weapons', *New Statesman and Society*, 1 December, pp. 24-5.

Beck, E. et al. (1987), 'HIV Testing', *British Medical Journal*, vol. 295.

Berridge, V. and Strong, P. (1990), 'No One Knew Anything: Some Issues in British AIDS Policy', in, Aggleton, P. et al., *AIDS: Individual, Cultural and Policy Dimensions*, Falmer Press, London, pp. 233-52.

Campbell, J. and Waters, W. (1987), 'Public Knowledge about AIDS increasing', *British Medical Journal*, vol. 294.

DHSS (Department of Health and Social Security) (1987), *AIDS: Monitoring response to the public education campaign*, HMSO, London.

DoH (Department of Health) (1989), *AIDS: Response by the Government to the 7th Report from the Social Services Committee Session*, Cm 925, HMSO, London.

Fumento, M. (1990), *The Myth of Heterosexual AIDS*, Basic Books, New York.

Garland, R. (1987), 'AIDS - the British Context', *Health Education Journal*, vol. 46, pp. 50-2.

HEA (Health Education Authority) (1989), *AIDS Programme: First Annual Report*, HEA, London.

HEA (1990), *AIDS and Sexual Health Programme: Summary of Second Annual Report* HEA, London.

Kapila, M. and Wellings, K. (1987), *The UK Public Education Campaign*, HEA, London.

Kirp, D. and Bayer, R. (eds) (1992), *AIDS in the Industrialized Democracies*, Rutgers University Press, New York.

Klein, R. and Day, P. (1990), 'Interpreting the Unexpected; the Case of AIDS Policy Making in Britain', *Journal of Public Policy*, vol. 9.

Naylor, W. (1985), 'Walking Time Bomb', *Medicine in Society*, vol. 11, pp. 5-10.

Nutbeam, D. et al., (1989), 'Public Knowledge and Attitudes to AIDS', *Public Health*, vol. 103.

Orr, A. (1989), 'Legal AIDS, implications of AIDS and HIV for British and American Law', *Journal of Medical Ethics*, vol. 15.

Schramm-Evans, Z. (1990), 'AIDS: Responses 1986-7', University of London, Unpublished PhD. Thesis.

SSSC (Social Services Select Committee)(1989), *AIDS*, 202, HMSO, London.

SSSC (1987), *Problems Associated with AIDS*, vol. ii, 182-II, HMSO, London.

Street, J. and Weale, A. (1992), 'Britain: Policy-Making in a Hermetically Sealed System', in, Kirp, D. and Bayer, R. (eds), *AIDS in the Industrialized Democracies*, Rutgers University Press, New York, pp. 185-220.

Weeks, J. (1981), *Sex, Politics and Society*, Longman, London.

Wiseman, D. and Bodell, D. (1990), 'Sustaining Safer Sex', *AIDS Dialogue*, vol. 4.

Young, H. (1990), *One of Us*, Pan, London.

6 The failure to implement an anti-smoking policy

Melvyn D. Read

This chapter examines the failure of successive British governments to adopt tough measures against the tobacco industry in favour of a preventive health strategy. I begin by showing that certain sections of the British public show an increase in the number of cigarettes smoked and that a recent study indicates that the majority of the public is in favour of a ban on smoking in public places. Despite these findings, which support earlier studies, government remains unwilling to take a pro-active approach to the smoking-health controversy. I then show that government policy has adopted a 'victim blaming' strategy which emphasises the crucial role of the individual in prevention. In doing so, certain assumptions are made about individual beliefs and actions. However, such assumptions may be erroneous. Greater attention must be given to influences on life-styles particularly those external pressures which people find so difficult to resist.

Having considered the problems of policy making inherent within the health-smoking arena I then go on to examine the policies which are in place. I show that successive British governments have consistently refuted the idea of using legislation to constrain the tobacco industry. Instead, they have preferred to use codes of practice which manifest themselves in voluntary agreements; an approach which was underpinned by economic considerations.

Having established that there is an economic dependency I propose that much of the government's response favouring prevention is a consequence of increasing opposition to the tobacco industry. The failure of government to adopt serious anti-smoking policies has resulted in a shift in the activities of certain charities. The evidence indicates that these charities are providing funds to assist those involved in the area of preventive smoking-related policies.

In order to combat the growing opposition I argue that the tobacco industry has developed a series of networks designed to promote its advertising activities. I look at those groups which make up the various networks, paying particular attention to the importance of sponsorship. Then I consider the support that cigarette manufacturers can call on in the House of Commons. I show that this support has several dimensions, can cross party boundaries and that the very highest political offices have been supportive of the tobacco industry.

I conclude that there is fundamental support for the tobacco industry. While an economic dimension ensures governmental approval I argue that the support has many facets with much depending on sponsorship. Through this financial backing relationships develop to underscore the activities of the tobacco industry. Moreover, the industry can also rely upon a number of MPs who will oppose any legislative proposals designed to restrict advertising activities. Consequently, we can argue that ideological considerations take priority over health imperatives.

Smoking - evidence, attitudes and debates

The list of diseases attributable to smoking has increased quite dramatically (DHSS, 1989). Recent estimates suggest that smoking is responsible for about 110,000 deaths each year in Great Britain; 17 per cent of all deaths (Johnson et al., 1991). 17 per cent of women and 27 per cent of men who smoke regularly will die before they reach 65 years. For nonsmokers, the comparable figure is 13 per cent (Johnson et al, 1991, p. 12). These figures understate the problem. They do not take account for those made ill by passive smoking or the impact of smoking on maternal and infant health.

British Social Attitudes; The 8th Report, (Ben-Shlomo et al., 1992) shows that the number of smokers is in decline but some population groups are experiencing an upturn. Young women below the age of 35 years are particularly susceptible. Smoking among the working-classes and the less qualified is more prevalent than among the middle-classes and the better educated (1992, p. 157).

People are aware of the dangers associated with smoking. In the survey, three out of five respondents said they would try to give up smoking within the next two years. Interestingly, young men rather than young women want to stop smoking. 87 per cent of respondents gave health as the most important reason for stopping. Cost (51 per cent) and family pressure (43 per cent) were the next most reported reasons. Women were more likely to cite social pressures for giving up cigarettes. However, social reasons seemed to have little overall impact of the decision to discontinue with the habit (1992, p.159-60).

Respondents perceived passive smoking, exposure to other people's tobacco smoke, as dangerous. 75 per cent of men under 35 years, and 84 per cent of women agreed that proximity to cigarette smoke was 'risky'. Existing smokers seemed less concerned about the dangers (1992, p.164). In all, 63 per cent of respondents, who smoked, admitted that other people smoking in public places had bothered them (1992, p.165). The report concludes that a large majority of the public favour restricting or banning smoking in public places (1992, p. 169).

Such strong evidence should strengthen the argument of those who seek to implement anti-smoking policy. However, the development of policies in the health-smoking controversy must overcome fundamental ideological obstacles (Calnan, 1984). The debate focuses on the extent to which the role of the state involves regulating both individual smoking behaviour and the activities of the tobacco industry. Smoking, it argues, should be a matter of personal choice and such choices can be made only if the individual has sufficient information to make the most rational choice. With relevant information about the inherent health risks of a particular action then, and only then, can individuals make proper decisions about the cost and benefits of their actions. But this argument ignores the aggressive, persuasive activities of diverse and powerful agencies and those ideologies which underpin the vested interest of those agencies. On the one hand, the Department of Health (DoH) battles to create an awareness and an environment which encourages individuals to change their behaviour. On the other hand, some Departments are engaged with developing policies which directly promote those industrial interests which threaten individual and public health. Government must accommodate these competing and conflicting interests.

An ideological position underpins both individual freedoms and industrial activity. Anti-smoking campaigners recognise no half measures. They wish to expunge the existence of tobacco completely. In contrast, those who campaign on health issues in other areas tend to seek moderation in behaviour, for example, less salt or no more than 21 units of alcohol a week. Others may demand changes in the method of production. Rarely is the campaign for abolition of both a product and the manufacturing industry. Anti-smoking campaigners, then, face stiff opposition from tobacco manufacturers and from those who defend an ideological position. These defendants contend that the onus it on individuals to make their own decisions, without interference from the heavy hand of the state.

Such an argument is tenable only if external influences on individuals to behave in a particularly hazardous way are not significantly greater than those which promote the opposite cause. For instance, the tobacco industry spends vast sums promoting not only the product but also the image of the cigarette manufacturers. The resources available to the industry are well in excess of those available to anti-smoking campaigners. The expenditure of these resources enables the industry to be portrayed as both caring and of benefit to society. It also presents a somewhat glamorous and sophisticated image. Such external influences are difficult to overcome. Below I shall look at some of the persuasive methods used by the industry.

Government responses

Underlying these external influences and, in part, explaining the failure of government to adopt a more aggressive attitude towards the tobacco companies is the economic value which the Exchequer derives from tobacco. Friedman has rightly identified the economic and political importance of tobacco which is based upon taxation (Friedman, 1975). The importance of revenue, then, may go some way to explaining why, despite the government's stated intention to improve the health of the nation, so little has been done. In 1991, *The Health of the Nation* identified smoking as the most important cause of ill health and disability. In 1992, the emphasis of *The Health of the Nation* had switched the focus of health care from the process, the type of treatment provided by doctors, to the success of treatment measured by the number of lives saved. The government had set itself a target to reduce cigarette sales by 40 per cent while resisting all demands for a ban on tobacco advertising.

The white paper stated that successive governments had effectively controlled tobacco advertising by voluntary agreements. It declared that:

> This Government believes that such agreement continues to represent the best way of controlling tobacco advertising, but recognizes that there is widespread concern that such controls should be strong and effective. It therefore proposes to review the effects of tobacco advertising, particularly on children, and consider what further steps are necessary (DHSS, 1992).

Critics argued that the government target was 'hypocritical' without an advertising ban (Brindle and Mihill, 1992). Virginia Bottomley, Secretary of State for Health, stated that the government would press for an end to European Community (EC) subsidies for tobacco growing. At home anti-smoking policy would continue much as before. It would be a combination of maintaining a price deterrent through taxation, education programmes and the voluntary agreements on tobacco advertising.

There seems little new on offer for rarely has legislation been considered. The Act of Parliament which prohibited the sale of cigarettes to children was passed in 1933. This Act was strengthened in 1986 by the *Protection of Children Act* which was enacted to stop Skoal Bandits being sold to children. In 1965 a ban on all cigarette advertising on Independent Television was introduced. This was extended to commercial radio in 1973. Other statutes have included anti-smoking measures: the 1965 *Food and Drugs Act*; the 1970 *Food Hygiene (General) Regulations* and the *Transport Act* which allowed British Rail to prohibit smoking in some parts of its trains. Indeed, carriages where smoking in permitted on British Rail are now the exception rather than the rule. Such prohibitions have been extended for safety reasons to London's Underground. Some airlines have introduced flights which do not permit smoking at all. Although these measures go some way to dealing with the smoking-health dimension of the preventive health issue, it is clear that legislation has never been seriously considered as a weapon against the tobacco industry.

The preferred method of regulation has always been voluntary agreements - the lynch pin of government's campaign against smoking. Between 1945 and 1971 the government and the tobacco industry concentrated on areas where they found agreement. Much of the research into smoking related diseases was funded by the Tobacco Manufacturing Select Committee. This was set up in 1956 and became the Tobacco Research Council (TRC) in 1963. The influence gained by the tobacco industry was enormous. David Horn, director of the National Clearinghouse for Smoking and Health in the United States of America, said of the TRC:

> Though supported by the tobacco industry, its statistics are relied on, and used by the government. The efforts of the council seem to be directed more to solving the problem than denying it exists (cited in Fritschler, 1983, p.134).

The British government adopted a two pronged smoking policy. It publicised the hazards of smoking generally and campaigned to persuade young people not to smoke. There was little evidence to suggest that government was prepared to take more aggressive actions. Indeed, in 1971 the Royal College of Physicians (RCP) reported:

> ... that Ministers, while accepting the evidence ... are guided in
> their actions by the view that the risks are regrettable but
> inevitable consequences of a habit which they believe to be an
> essential source of revenue (RCP, 1971, p.21).

On 2 February 1971, the Prime Minister announced an interdepartmental review of the report from the RCP (HC, vol.810, col.346, 2 February 1971). The unpublished report shows that the government was cautious. It was proposed to wait and see if the new agreement would have any effect upon smoking behaviour. Furthermore, it was decided to give less emphasis to the hazards of smoking (Phillips, 1980).

History was repeating itself. In 1951 Iain McCleod, Minister of Health, a recent convert to an anti-smoking ethos, was compelled to accept the Treasury's view regarding the value of tobacco as a source of revenue. The interdepartmental Committee called for a balance between human needs and economic fact; the future cost to the Exchequer was a significant factor in the balancing act. A sharp decline in smoking would add significantly to the pensions bill by the year 2001 as more people would live to pensionable age. It was estimated that with a fall of 20 per cent in cigarette consumption the Exchequer would suffer a net loss of about £155 million in tax revenue. This compared the loss in excise duty with the gain accruing from the additional purchase tax associated with extra consumer spending.

By 1971 the connection between smoking and certain diseases could no longer be ignored. As if to pre-empt the RCP's report, representatives of the industry met with the Secretary of State for Social Services and officials of the Department of Health and Social Security (DHSS) and the Department of Trade and Industry. They agreed to incorporate an health warning from H.M. Government that 'smoking can damage your health' in the design of all cigarette packets sold in the United Kingdom. Press and poster advertising would carry similar warnings. In addition, it was decided to appoint a scientific committee to monitor research into the use of tobacco and substitute materials. However, the committee's findings were not to be made widely available. It would be provided to properly accredited researchers only and then on a confidential basis (HC Debates, vol.816, col.211-2, 29 April 1971).

Attention was beginning to focus on the relationship between government and the tobacco industry. In the wake of the interdepartmental meeting it was agreed to draw up a code of practice. At the request of the Secretary of State for Social Services, the cigarette manufacturers, represented by the Tobacco Advisory Council (TAC), agreed that all packets of cigarettes produced by them for the UK trade should carry a government health warning. However, the manufacturers also had the following statement inserted into the code:

> The manufactures undertake themselves to ensure that the Code
> of Practice is observed in the Spirit as well as the letter.

This gave the tobacco industry immense control because it ensured that they were subject to self-regulation.

The industry was fortunate to gain this degree of self-regulation. It is clear that this type of agreement constrained the government's ability to manoeuvre, particularly in the health-smoking controversy. Difficulties were amplified by the fact that no less than three codes of practice have been put into operation. The *Tobacco Products Advertising and Promotion and Health Warnings* was established in 1970 and is monitored by the DoH. It regulates both the form and quality of tobacco advertising together with the display of health warnings on cigarette packets. The DoH also oversees the *Tobacco Product Modification and Research* code of practice which is concerned with reducing tar levels in cigarettes. Clearly, the aims of the department conflict with those of the tobacco industry.

The Department of the Environment (DoE) oversees *Sports Sponsorship and Advertising*. The two government departments differ in their approach. While the DoH opposes cigarette promotion the DoE actively encourages it, particularly to sport and the arts. The industry is much less constrained in this area so there is less conflict. Sports sponsorship is one of the more potent forms of advertising. It offers both direct selling and that touch of glamour with which tobacco companies seek to associate their products. The arts provides that touch of sophistication and social acceptability. Officials from the DoH attend discussions between the tobacco industry and the DoE, but they cannot participate directly.

The codes of practice allow for the imposition of progressively tougher restrictions on the promotional activities of the tobacco industry. However, this is not a one way process by any means. Having established the ground rules the cigarette manufacturers find ingenious methods to circumvent them. Despite this, they maintain that they operate within both the letter and spirit of the agreements. Voluntary agreements, then, legitimate the promotional activities of the industry.

More importantly, self regulation cemented over cracks which began to develop in the close relationship between government and the tobacco industry. The first major threat occurred in 1974 when David Owen, Under Secretary at the Department of Health, threatened to use the *Medicines Act, 1968,* to control tobacco (Sherwood, 1975, p.369). The industry agreed to stop advertising free samples but refused to comply with demands to discontinue using gift coupons. One year later, Owen was forced to tell the House of Commons that he had written to the industry telling them that its response was not acceptable (HC Debates, vol.895, col.317, 8 July 1975).

The voluntary agreements, then, seemed to offer no effective means of constraining the industry's promotional activities. Other means had to be found but the manufactures adopted a more arms length approach to government. Only in the last resort would they participate. Indeed, the industry refused outright to concede on the issue of gift coupons which they saw as the most direct and effective advertising tool in the battle for increased market share.

Despite the increasing reluctance of cigarette manufacturers to negotiate, relations with government never deteriorated beyond the threat of legislation. Indeed, once David Owen moved to the Foreign Office, government ministers became more supportive of the tobacco industry.

The voluntary agreements, introduced in response to the RCP's Report of 1971, were more of an inconvenience than a restraint on the tobacco industry. Every three years or so the industry was expected to concede more and more restrictions from which opponents could assess the industry's compliance with the codes of practice. As the decade drew to a close little had been achieved. The tobacco industry continued to promote its products with impunity by circumventing the codes of practice, but in a way which was legitimated by government. Yet, successive Ministers have consistently pointed to these agreements as indicators of their activity in the area of health and smoking.

Anti-smoking groups

The close of the decade saw tobacco industry increasingly under pressure from external opposition. The economic argument, underpinned by tax revenue, was no longer sufficient to justify smoking. Health was becoming an important part of the equation. The RCP's report of 1971 had been instrumental in instituting voluntary agreements but, more importantly, it saw the establishment of Action on Smoking and Health (ASH). Born out of frustration at being unable to resolve the smoking problem, ASH was designed to mobilise and coordinate voluntary action against smoking (RCP, 1977, p. 27). The aim was to promote a series of related projects designed to raise public and government awareness about the dangers of smoking.

Initially ASH received a government grant of £25,000: this funding has continued. Recently the work undertaken by ASH has been in conjunction with other major charities. Four influential charities including; the British Heart Foundation (BHF), the Imperial Cancer Research Fund (ICRF), the Cancer Research Campaign (CRC) and the Chest, Heart and Stroke Association (CHSA), have adopted a more positive approach to prevention.

The BHF was set up in 1961 to provide funds for research into heart disease; principally to support basic research into the causes of coronary heart disease. Increasingly, the Foundation has been active in educating both the medical profession and the public using both lectures and publications. In 1984, *Guide-lines on Reducing the Risk of a Heart Attack* called for changes in lifestyles within the community as a whole. The emphasis was on persuading children to adopt healthier living. Parents were encouraged to lead by example; to change their behaviour not for the sake of their children alone but also for the good of their own health.

The shift towards prevention was even more noteworthy when the Foundation urged the government to endorse the recommendations of the World Health Organization Expert Committee's *Community Prevention and Control of Cardiovascular Diseases* (WHO, 1986). The main advice was to formulate a national plan for preventing and controlling disease by setting out a series of achievable goals. It pointed out that the occurrence of disease was often influenced by the decisions of government departments and agencies which base decisions on economic or political grounds. The Foundation recognised that it could not work in isolation but should work in coordination with other groups working in this area. In doing so they should oppose the activities of the powerful vested interests.

The ICRF, founded in 1902, is the principal fund-raiser for research into cancer and funds are drawn from the public in the form of voluntary contributions. These funds maintain scientific staff and laboratories but also provide grants for research departments at various hospitals. Its main work is at the secondary and tertiary levels of prevention with scant attention to primary prevention. However, the value of prevention has been recognised in recent years. Each year about 2 per cent of the charity's funds are allocated to preventive research.

The CRC, set up in 1923 as the British Empire Cancer Campaign, is a body which raises funds for particular projects. In 1967 following an initiative by medical practitioners the charity and the Medical Research Council (MRC) came together (*The Times*, 10 April 1967). The MRC had found a new source of funds while the CRC found that it had acquired a new status.

Research funded by CRC tends to be concentrated in areas of high technology. This, means that such research is often at the very frontier of technological advancement. Given the constraints imposed by the limitations of technology, examination of the social and economic conditions associated with cancer is one way forward. The CRC has adopted a view that preventing cancer is one of its main objectives. Success is possible only when factors which cause or increase risks are known.

Since the majority of adolescents who try smoking become dependent upon tobacco, young people should be dissuaded from taking up the habit. Consequently, the charity's preventive strategy tends to be aimed at the young. The CRC is unable to take individual action against smoking because it lacks both the techniques and resources to do so. It takes part in events such as National No Smoking Days which are designed to develop public awareness of the dangers of smoking. These events also provide an opportunity for non-campaigning organisations to participate in social and political actions.

In contrast, prevention is high on the priority list of the Chest, Heart and Stroke Association; its public activities involve producing publications about coronary heart disease prevention. It has adopted a course of action which focuses on primary health care and offers support to primary health care teams. In 1982 it funded the Oxford Prevention of Heart Attack and Stroke Project. This programme has been successful in defining the scope for prevention and allows general practitioners (GPs) to engage in prevention without disrupting their practice and at minimal cost.

This changing role has occurred, in part, because successive governments have opted for voluntary agreements or have resorted to moral exhortation. This half measure approach is preferred to legislation and improving education and information dissemination. Lesley Doyal points out that these contradictions are put into sharp relief when annual government expenditure on publicising the hazards of smoking is compared with the amount spent by the tobacco industry annually on advertising and sponsorship of sport and the arts (Doyal, 1983, p. 83).

Until the late 1970s it was clear that government priorities were also reflected by the various British cancer research organisations. In 1979 both the CRC and ICRC spent about 2 per cent of annual income on educational or preventive projects. The 'prestige medical projects' aimed at finding a cure for cancer attracted the largest proportion of resources. Over time this position has changed. First, advances have been made in understanding the nature of cancer. As a consequence, resources are being allocated towards examining lifestyles, smoking, alcohol, diet and physical exercise (*BMJ*, 22 December 1979, p. 1610). Secondly, the research charities now recognise that individual political impotency can be overcome by combining their interest in prevention to become more effective and wide-ranging in their activities. Third, the charitable status of these organisations has acted as a constraint on their ability to campaign publicly or apply political pressure. They may prevail by working with other groups whose skills lie not with medical research but in campaigning both politically and publicly. Thus the scientific establishment, the professionals and the campaigners can present a united front which government will find difficult to ignore.

Industry responses

In the light of these changing circumstances, the tobacco industry has been forced into adopting a more acceptable public image. Instead of relying on the simple 'economic' relationship which has developed between the manufacturers and the Treasury the industry has sought to establish links with other departments. The one resource which the tobacco industry has in abundance is money. In the late 1970s financial sponsorship became the most potent method of advertising available to manufactures. The major advantage was that smokers and non-smokers benefited equally.

Jeremy Bullmore, when Deputy Chairman of J. Walter Thompson, defined advertising as: 'Any paid-for communication intended to inform and/or influence one or more people (Bullmore, 1976, p.1). He proposed that without advertising certain cigarette brands and reputations would suffer owing to 'the inevitable attrition in public awareness due to the passage of time' and 'because the public mind itself is always changing (Bullmore, 1976, p. 5).

Sponsorship offered cigarette manufacturers the opportunity to circumvent many of the restrictions which were imposed upon their advertising activities by the codes of practice on advertising. Initially this tactic was adopted in response to the television and radio and, subsequently, cinema ban on advertising. The advantage of sponsorship is that it provides an attractive means of promoting a product. It is often associated with health and fitness, thereby countering the negative images of cigarettes presented by anti-smoking campaigners. Sponsorship creates a positive image among the public particularly when certain types of events are chosen. Glamorous or highly popular sports, such as motor racing and cricket are obvious targets. They have a high media profile, especially with the BBC, thereby receiving television coverage which is in contravention of the Television Act (1964).

Barrie Gill, Chief Executive of Championship Sports Specialists Ltd., told Peter Taylor that an event like motor racing was an ideal sport for sponsorship:

> It's got glamour and world-wide television coverage. It's a ten-month activity involving sixteen races in fourteen countries with drivers of sixteen nationalities. After football its the number one multi-national sport. It's got total global exposure, total global hospitality, total media coverage and 600 million people watching it on TV every fortnight (cited in Taylor, 1984, p. 101-2).

Costs seem high but when compared to launching a new cigarette brand they are quite small (Taylor, 1984, p. 103). In an attempt to assess the commercial costs of advertising through sporting events on television it has been shown that the costs to tobacco manufactures would be in the region of £60,000 for every hour of broadcast snooker. For British motor sport this figure would rise to £510,000 for each hour (Adheath Ltd, 1992, p.14). Consequently, even £500,000 spent on one event is good practice. With worldwide distribution, sponsorship probably offers the companies very good value for money indeed.

At a more fundamental level sponsorship creates an environment in which personal networks among the more influential members of society and Ministers can be nurtured. Some departments rely on sponsorship to provide much needed financial assistance which would otherwise be provided by government. While the DoE is the most obvious example even the DoH has accepted money from the tobacco industry for medical research.

As shown earlier, sponsorship offers a simple and cheap means of getting round the ban which prohibits cigarettes being advertised on television. The government's position on sponsorship is plain. Neil Macfarlane told the House of Commons that:

> The Government's aim and policy remain to maintain a balance between the vital sponsorship that our sport today needs whilst ensuring that the voluntary agreement is kept and there is thus no excessive advertising of tobacco in the sensitive environment of sporting events.
>
> I am deeply anxious to ensure that all tobacco companies and their representatives ensure that breaches do not occur. If they do occur, I need to be told immediately and I guarantee that they will not occur again (HC Debates, vol.44, col.802, 30 June 1983).

This position was re-iterated by Richard Tracey, the Parliamentary Under-Secretary of State for the Environment, three years later when the code of practice was up for discussion. Concern was expressed about the level of television exposure which cigarettes received and the DoH was keen to change the existing rules. Advice was being taken from the medical professions and other agencies including the Health Education Council (HEC) and the Sports Council, two bodies financed by government. The Sports Council declared its opposition to tobacco sponsorship in principle but accepted funding because the operating code of practice legitimated sponsorship.

The HEC was in flux; it was about to become the Health Education Authority (HEA) and the new director, Ann Burdus, had a commercial interest in tobacco advertising, although this was never known to have affected her work for the HEA (Veitch and Hencke, 1987). This position was compounded by the decision of the DoH to accept an £11 million grant, from the tobacco industry, for research purposes. It was no surprise when the Minister told the House of Commons:

> The voluntary system remains the most effective method of restricting and controlling the impact of the tobacco industry's sponsorship of sport. We consider that legislation is not needed … Tobacco sponsorship is now below 10 per cent of all sports sponsorship (HC Debates, vol.92, col. 644, 21 February 1986).

This fails to take into account that tobacco sponsorship concentrates on events which receive the greatest media attention. Financial support is not distributed equally among sports

Sponsorship of the arts confers respectability on both product and industry. Crucially, it gives valuable access to influential individuals and institutions. Indeed, sponsorship of the arts serves at least three purposes. First, it presents the manufacturers as public benefactors, an historical role which they have always played. Second, it allows access to non-tobacco related institutions and government departments which enhances the creation of personal and industrial networks for the benefit of the tobacco industry. Third, it underpins the government's attitude to sectors like the arts, highlighting the need for self-sufficiency.

Sir Roy Strong, Director of the Victoria and Albert Museum, argued that:

> Our basic existence will continue, of course, to be secured by government but growth and development will have to spring henceforth from sponsorship, the realization of our commercial potential and persuading our visitors to dig even deeper into their pockets. The financial swing has certainly sharpened our focus (Strong, 1986).

Three years later the Arts Council took the matter of serious underfunding directly to the Prime Minister, by-passing the Arts Minister, Richard Luce. Luke Rittner, the Council's Secretary General, warned that the arts were facing disaster (*The Guardian*, 18 July 1989, p. 3). Luce, responded to the pleas for additional funding by pointing to sponsorship:

> Museums are free to operate such schemes under present arrangements and there is nothing to stop them moving in that direction (HC Debate, vol. 157 , col. 14, 18 July 1989).

The increasing financial support of sport and arts is one indication that the relationship between the tobacco industry and government was under threat. In 1980, the manufactures had acceded to government demands in the belief that a commitment to anti-smoking legislation was to be included in the Queen's speech. The agreement contained additional restrictions on advertising expenditures. The most significant feature of the new agreement was that it would last twenty months rather than an expected four years. On expiration of the short agreement the DoH would introduce legislation.

Health Ministers, Patrick Jenkin and Sir George Young, intended to use the *Health Services (Miscellaneous Provisions) Bill* to introduce legislation. This proposal was accepted by the Cabinet's Legislative sub-committee in November 1980. Patrick Jenkin told the House of Commons that he had:

> ... made it clear to the industry that the House must be free to continue to express its view on smoking and initiate such action as it might see fit; but I have indicated to the industry that I can give no undertaking on behalf of the government to obstruct

legislation in the meantime (HC Debate, vol.992, col. 124, 21 November 1980).

However, the Leader of the House, Francis Pym, threw out the proposal owing to pressure of time on the Commons.

Meanwhile, the Health Ministers applied pressure to the Sports Minister calling for tougher action with the tobacco industry. However, the Health Department had no control over sport sponsorship and successive Sports Ministers have successfully resisted demands for the imposition of greater restrictions on sponsorship.

In 1981, following a cabinet reshuffle, the health team was dispersed. Sir George Younger was moved to Environment, Russell Fairgrieve returned to the back-benches with a knighthood and Patrick Jenkin was promoted to Secretary of State at the Department of Industry. Gerard Vaughan was eventually replaced by Kenneth Clarke, in March 1982. Clarke, an MP for Nottingham, with a constituency interest in tobacco, was consistently predisposed towards the tobacco industry.

Whilst the general links between government and the tobacco industry were weakening, the industry was establishing close links elsewhere. At the same time, anti-smoking groups were beginning to present a united opposition to the existing links.

Producer networks and the policy community

What seems clear, then, is that the link between government and industry had been very strong; sufficiently strong to constitute a policy community. Following Rhodes (1983, p. 73-4), I have been able to identify: shared general interest, exclusive membership, horizontal inter-dependence together with extensive exchanges of information and considerable formal and informal contact, and an externalised structure (see Read, 1992).

The most important feature of this policy community is that it is supported by an external structure which may be defined as a producer network. This is distinguished by the prominent role played by industrial interests in policy making. In these networks, the industrial actor promotes self interest, intervening only where a 'particular' interest is threatened. Such producers tend to distance themselves from general politics although they may be involved with general industrial associations; for example, the CBI.

However, industry does maintain autonomy of action and political and economic pressure can be exerted on the decision making process. The government's dependence on tobacco was explained, by Sir David Nicholson (Euro MP and Chairman of Rothman International) in terms of 'one of the prime activities of this industry (being) in effect to act as a tax collector for the government concerned'. Indeed, the tobacco industry was considered to be an important element in the government's strategy for defeating inflation. Speaking of the tobacco industry, Leon Brittain, argued:

> monetary and fiscal restraint remain essential to the success of
> the Government's strategy of defeating inflation and thereby
> securing the condition for substantial growth of output and

employment.

He continued:

> Shifting the balance in favour of industry and against the
> consumer is a shift in direction that the Government think it
> reasonable to take (HC Debates, vol.8, col. 72-75, 6 July
> 1986).

While an increase in indirect taxation seems to threaten the tobacco industry, perversely it underscores the economic importance of tobacco. Increases in excise duty exposes the anti-smoking campaign as a potential threat to both the industry and the country.

However, the impact of the general health message, within the country, illustrates the extent of the challenge that the industry faces. Putting the economy before public health is now open to question. To allay concern, tobacco manufacturers must demonstrate both a general economic importance and a social value. To establish that link the industry must bring together groups which represent both the economic and social sectors.

The economic sector consists of those groups which are economically effective. These will be organisations from the distributive trades, employees representatives, particularly the Tobacco Workers Union and unions associated with the distributive trades, and the media. Those organisations representing society tend to be drawn from the sponsored sector, for example, the arts and sports. Clearly, government departments are incorporated into one or other of these groups depending upon their brief. Some departments might prefer to remain 'neutral' but neutrality contributes to the nurturing of the industry because they are then incorporated into the network of industry interests. This approach enables the tobacco industry to absorb government departments who are potentially antagonistic. The function of this network, then, is to protect the interests the tobacco industry and it does so, where there is correspondence of interest between groups and the industry itself. Of course, there is conflict on occasion but the general coincidence of interest is recognised.

At the heart of the network is a 'core' or policy community consisting of the government and the tobacco industry. External to this central core is the producer network, a structure which includes those groups most able to fully serve the interests of the manufacturers. In effect, this network emphasises the benefits which accrue to society from the tobacco industry and this underscores the link with government through sponsorship. The advertising industry has become a significant actor in this area. Not only does it participate through sponsorship but it also promotes the tobacco products in such a way that the public are vulnerable to the messages of the manufacturers. Attention was drawn to this function by John Havard, Secretary to the British Medical Association (BMA), when he said that:

> It is clear that young non-smokers and experimental smokers is
> the single most important group which should be protected
> from cigarette advertising ... We are now able to present

> further evidence which shows that the tobacco industry is ...
> directly reaching these susceptible target groups through the
> pages of women's magazines (Jacobson and Amos, 1985, p.2).

One advantage of having the advertising industry within the network is that it operates in two directions at one time. First, it applies additional pressure on government by stressing the financial importance of the industry and highlighting each area where tobacco money is important. Second, it links those interests which are external to the producer network but still play a crucial role in supporting the advertising and promotional needs of the industry. Clearly, the most crucial and, perhaps, most influential group is the media. Without assistance from the media, both newspaper and broadcast, the promotion of tobacco products, through sponsorship for example, would be much more difficult.

Most newspapers take cigarette advertisements and it is estimated that tobacco advertising provides about 10 per cent of income. So, it is in the interests of publishers to ensure the survival of the tobacco trade. There is conflict however. Manufacturers have been known to use their veto power over publishers, by temporarily removing advertisements from particular publications where articles highly critical of the industry have been published (Hird, 1981, p. 6). Such a move on the part of manufacturers is frequently more of a rebuke than a punitive measure.

Unions and the retail and distributive trades provide support by lobbying on a number of fronts, particularly employment. Christine Godfrey and Geoffrey Hardman (1987) have shown that the number of people employed in the tobacco industry has declined significantly in recent years. However, they highlight the fact that job losses in this industry were a consequence of improved production methods and increased productivity.

Many other jobs are indirectly dependent upon tobacco in agriculture or in those industries supplying goods and machinery for the production process and in the distribution and retailing trades where the greatest number of indirectly dependent jobs can be found (Godfrey and Hardman, 1987, p. 1162). Citing the work of Mackay and Edwards (1982) Godfrey and Hardman suggest that in 1980 an additional 115,000 jobs were dependent on the retailing of tobacco. In times of high, and rising, levels of unemployment such arguments carry great weight.

These arguments, which underscore the relationships identified within a network, are no longer sufficient. If government adopted a more aggressive attitude to support preventive health policies then the tobacco industry would be subject to a much greater threat. What seems clear, then, is that there is overt political hindrance to prevention, particularly in the health-smoking issue. While government can do more, individual ministers and back-bench MPs can influence the degree of constraint imposed upon the tobacco industry.

Policy constraints

One of the most important influences has been that of individual back-bench MPs. Here, there is a tendency to stress the role of 'the tobacco lobby'. Whilst costly public relations firms are employed to promote the cigarette manufacturers two or three committed MPs are more cost effective. In 1981, a Private Members' Bill, *Tobacco Products (Control of Advertising, Sponsorship and Promotion)* was effectively opposed by Sir Anthony Kershaw (Conservative MP for Stroud) using accepted delaying tactics. However, it seems clear that the Private Members' Bill procedure would have prevented the Bill progressing further (Marsh and Read, 1986). The main point here is that two or three strategically placed supporters are an adequate deterrent to anti-tobacco campaigns and legislative proposals in the House of Commons.

This does not mean that we could not identify a body of MPs who would defend the interests of the tobacco industry. Certainly, with the huge number of commercial interests which are represented in the House of Commons, particularly among Conservative MPs, some will act as parliamentary consultants for the tobacco industry. Other MPs can be relied on to defend the tobacco industry on ideological grounds. Amongst these, some are opposed to using legislation to constrain industry in general. Mrs. Thatcher, recognised the hazards of smoking and that public opinion favoured a ban of tobacco advertising, but argued that: 'We in the UK have a tradition of proceeding by consent rather than legislation in such matters' (cited in, Cohen and Anderson, 1984, p.9).

Others use the ideological defence of freedom of choice and the freedom of the individual. This underpins the commitment of individual responsibility for one's own health. Indeed, a pledge to this form of prevention was used to explain the establishment of the Health Promotion Research Trust in 1981. This was a trust funded by the Tobacco industry but administered by the DoH. The only constraint on using the research funds was that none should be used to investigate smoking related diseases. At this stage, then, the DoH had been incorporated into the network which protects the tobacco industry.

Ideological constraints are not the prerogative of one party; they cross party boundaries. This was highlighted during the Ways and Means debate, *Tobacco Products*, which shifted the burden of tax away from petrol to tobacco (HC Debates, vol.8, col.72-138, 6 July 1981). Teddy Taylor (Conservative MP for Southend) defended the industry but also supported this increase in taxation on cigarettes. Tax increases were necessary for no reason other than: 'the simple principle that things should be paid for' (HC Debates, vol.8, col.81, 6 July 1981). He told the Labour Shadow Chancellor that these measures were a consequence of successive government's, particularly Labour governments, providing services for the community without charging the necessary tax for them.

Mr. Taylor made it clear that he had neither direct not indirect association with the companies. He described the tobacco industry as an: 'important industry with a record almost unique in British industry for coping with import penetration ... the tobacco industry achieved more in resisting imports and promoting exports ... provides good employment in so many areas where there is massive unemployment (or which) makes such a large contribution to the survival and prosperity of the small shops' (HC Debates, vol.8, col.84, 6 July 1981).

Peter Shore (Labour MP for Stepney and Poplar), stated that the Opposition was opposed to measures that would increase unemployment and reduce expenditure in the community. This concern was shared by Harvey Proctor (Conservative MP for Basildon), who, like Mr Shore, had a constituency interest. He defended the industry because:

> ... the large and unprecedented increase in tobacco taxes, with
> the inevitable drop in consumption of tobacco products, will
> have serious consequences for the United Kingdom tobacco
> industry (HC Debates, vol.8, col.89, 6 July 1981).

Constituency concern was raised again by Michael Martin (Labour MP for Glasgow, Springburn) an elected Member for 'an area in which unemployment is worsening day by day'. He argued that: 'The anti-smoking campaigners should be aware that though smoking can be harmful to one's health unemployment is harmful to both the individual and the family' (HC Debates, vol.8, col.86, 6 July 1981).

Unemployment was raised time and time again. Denis Canavan (Labour MP for West Stirlingshire) pointed out that the Stirling travel-to-work area, which served the tobacco factory there, had been singled out by the Secretary of State for Industry and relegated from development area status. Michael English (Conservative MP for Nottingham West) drew attention to the fact that two hundred employees at the John Player factory in Raleigh were working a two day week.

Labour MPs expressed concern about those most affected by an increase in taxation. Austen Mitchell (Labour MP for Grimsby) was fearful for those people who smoked; those looking for work and the less well off. Moves to cut smoking through fiscal measure smacked of the school ma'am (HC Debates, vol.8, col. 115, 6 July 1981). Dennis Skinner (Labour MP for Bolsover) continued this line of attack: 'It would be pensioners who would be most affected by increases in the price of tobacco ... It was no more than an attack on the working classes'.

What seems clear then is that there really is no real need for a large organised group to promote the interests of the tobacco industry. As we have seen above, support for the cigarette manufacturers cuts across party boundaries. More importantly, this championing hinges on at least four issues; the role of the MP as a consultant, ideological constraints, the constituency interest, and employment. The last three dimensions are important when defending the industry against potentially harmful legislative proposals or fiscal increases.

In recent years, the tobacco industry has found patronage at the highest political level. As a backbencher, Kenneth Clarke had defended the tobacco industry. He argued:

> ... the well being of the area which I represent is very much
> affected by the well being of the tobacco industry ... I can
> understand exasperation growing on the part of the tobacco
> industry, which is manufacturing a lawful product (HC
> Debates, vol. 905, col. 858, 16 January 1976).

When he became Minister of Health he continued his defence. In 1984, he told a *Panorama* team that tobacco companies were allowed to advertise on TV through sport because:

> ... we have a free country and this is a legal product and there
> is a limit to the extent to which you can go in actually putting

legal bans on what, those who market a product, are free to do.

He maintained that what went on television was a problem for the BBC and IBA but not for the government.

More recently Mrs. Thatcher has been criticised by European cancer experts for her opposition to compulsory 'smoking kills' warnings on the front of cigarette packets. The Europe Against Cancer campaign urged the European Community (EC) Council of Ministers to ban tobacco sponsorship of sports and the arts. There was also a call for an end to all tobacco advertising by the end of 1989. Mrs. Thatcher opposed these moves and it was believed that she would have been willing to go to the European Court of Justice in order to maintain Britain's right to veto health directives from Brussels.

Michael Wood, honourary secretary of the Cancer Education Coordinating Group for the UK and Ireland, attacked the British-supported voluntary agreements with the tobacco industry (Ballentyne, 1989). Dr. Martin Raw, adviser to the BMA on tobacco and Europe, accused Mrs.Thatcher of 'breathtaking hypocrisy' in personally supporting the Europe Against Cancer programme while opposing proposals to put it into practice. He stated that the European Commission had expected a rough ride from the tobacco industry for presenting these tobacco directives but had not expected the British government to do the industry's job (Raw, 1989).

British opposition to European proposals was not enough, however. On 11 February, 1992, the European Parliament voted to prohibit virtually all tobacco advertising throughout the Community. The vote rebuffed the largest and best financed lobbying campaign ever mounted by tobacco and advertising companies (Palmer, 1992). The final decision, to be made in November 1992, remains with the Council of Ministers but success in Strasbourg now seems likely. Nine of the twelve EC governments already favoured proposals which would allow advertising only at newsagents and specialist shops. Britain, Germany and Holland have opposed the measure and between them, present a possible block to approving the plan.

The British government's position was that the current voluntary code, with the tobacco companies now agreeing not to advertise in women's magazines, is more effective. As evidence it is claimed that the number of new smokers in Britain is lower than in countries where an advertising ban is enforced.

In July 1992 *The Sunday Times* revealed that (the now) Lady Thatcher is to become the international political consultant for Philip Morris, the world's biggest tobacco company. Her brief seems to be to assist the tobacco company to penetrate the tobacco markets of Eastern Europe and the Third World. In addition, she will help the company resist attempts to ban general tobacco advertising in the EC, to fight increases in cigarette taxes, and oppose state-run tobacco monopolies (Rufford et al., 1992). The report showed that Philip Morris had used the services of Lady Thatcher previously. An internal company memorandum dated March 31, 1992 stated: 'We have the ability to use Mrs Thatcher's services and skills over the next three years. On the few occasions we have asked for her advice, she has provided very skilful help'.

By considering this appointment, Lady Thatcher was condemned by Michael O'Connor, the civil servant in charge of tobacco policy from 1987 to 1989. He had written the speech which she had given to mark the start of Europe Against Cancer

Year. Because Lady Thatcher had a very high reputation in Eastern Europe it would be difficult to encourage them to resist the multinationals if she was batting for them. Mr. O'Connor, now the adviser to the World Health Organization on developing anti-tobacco policy in Eastern Europe, called upon John Major to reaffirm his support for health promotion and indicate that he would fight the tobacco industry (Watts, 1992).

Conclusion

What is clear, then, is that the tobacco industry has had governmental support at the very highest level. A Prime Minister, who was regarded as having almost absolute control over the Cabinet has demonstrated that she has no objection to the activities of the tobacco industry. This is in direct contrast to the position adopted when strongly supporting anti-smoking campaigns. We can only conjecture about her real views about prevention and the smoking-health controversy. Her recent consideration about working for the world's largest tobacco company indicate her real view on this issue.

Kenneth Clarke, an out spoken supporter of manufacturers, was Minister of Health for three years, 1982-1985. Perhaps we can see why the relationship between government and the tobacco industry has never been seriously threatened. Indeed, it goes some way to explain why the British government has consistently resisted attempts to prohibit advertising of tobacco. In fact, we might say that the 1980s has been one where the tobacco industry has enjoyed great support from very high political offices. Similarly, we do not need a conspiracy theory to explain why the tobacco industry receives support in the House of Commons. There are enough areas in which there is a coincidence of interests between the industry and a range of MP interests, that the industry can be assured of support both directly and indirectly.

The position of the tobacco industry as an employer, but also its careful and deliberate sponsorship in areas reliant upon extra-governmental funding, has allowed the industry to integrate itself not only into prestigious areas of advertising, but to augment its economic importance to the state as well. The advantages which naturally accrue to the tobacco industry from the tax revenues it produces, are multiplied when it can both provide research funding or subsidise government spending in the arts and sport. There are, as a consequence, formidable political, ideological and economic reasons why preventive health policies in the smoking policy area do not respond readily to efforts to reduce the levels of smoking-related disease.

Bibliography/references

Adheath Ltd. (1992), *Tobacco and the BBC: A review of how BBC TV promotes cigarettes through tobacco-sponsored sport,* Health Education Authority, London.

Ballentyne, A. (1989), 'PM attacked over stance on tobacco, *The Guardian,* 27 May.

Ben-Shlomo, Y., Sheiham, A. and Marmot, M. (1992), 'Smoking and Health', in, R. Jowell, et al., *British Social Attitudes: the 8th Report*, Dartmouth, Aldershot, pp.155-74.

Brindle, D. and Mihill, C. (1992), *The Guardian*. July 9, p.3.

British Heart Foundation (1984), *Guide-lines on Reducing the Risk of a Heart Attack*, British Heart Foundation, London.

Bullmore, J. (1976), *Advertising: What it is and what is it for?*, J. Walter Thompson, London.

Calnan, M. (1984), 'The Politics of Health: The case of smoking control', *Journal of Social Policy*, vol. 13, no. 3, pp.278-96.

Cohen, P. and Anderson, G. (1984), 'Smoke Screen', *New Statesman*, 9 March, pp.9-10.

DHSS (1976), *Prevention and Health, Everybody's Business*, HMSO, London

DHSS (1977), *Preventive Medicine*, vol. 1, report, HMSO, London.

DHSS (1986), *Preventive Medicine*, 44th Report from the Committee of Public Accounts, HMSO, London.

Department of Health (DoH) (1991), *Health of the Nation*, HMSO, London.

Doyal, L. (with I. Pennell) (1983), *The Political Economy of Health*, Pluto Press, London.

Friedman, K. M. (1975), *Public Policy and the Smoking-Health Controversy*, Lexington Books, New York.

Fritschler, A. L. (1983), *Smoking and Politics*, Prentice Hall, Englewood Hills.

Godfrey, C. and Hardman, G. (1987), 'Data Note-11. Employment in the U.K. Alcohol and Tobacco Industries', *British Journal of Addiction*, vol. 82, pp. 1157-67.

Hird, C. (1981), 'Taking on the tobacco men', *New Statesman*, 27 February.

Jacobson, B. and Amos, A. (1985), *When smoke gets in your eyes!*, BMA Professional Division and Health Education Council, London.

Johnson, K., Callum, C. and Killoran, A. (1991), *The Smoking Epidemic*, HEA, London.

MacKay, D.I. and Edwards, R.T. (1982), *The U.K. Tobacco Industry. Its Economic Significance*, PEIDA, Edinburgh.

Marsh, D. and Read, M. (1986), *Private Members' Bills*, Cambridge University Press, Cambridge.

Palmer, J. (1992), 'Euro-MPs vote for ban on tobacco advertising', *The Guardian*, 12 February 1992.

Phillips, M. (1980), *The Guardian*, 6 May.

Raw, M. (1989), *British Medical Journal*, 27 May.

Read, M. (1992), 'Policy Networks and Issue Networks: The Politics of Smoking', in, Marsh, D. and Rhodes, R.A.W. (eds), *Policy Networks and British Government*, Clarendon Press, Oxford.

Rhodes, R., Hardy, B. and Pudney, K. (1983), 'Constraints on the National Community of Local Government: Members, Other Governments and Policy Communities, *Discussion Paper 6*, Department of Government, University of Essex.

Royal College of Physicians (1971), *Smoking and Health Now*, Pitman, London.

Royal College of Physicians (1977), *Smoking or Health*, Pitman, London.

Rufford, N., Leppard, D. and Burrell, I. (1992), 'Thatcher gets $1m job with the top US tobacco firm', *The Sunday Times*, 19 July.

Sherwood, M. (1975), 'Smoking goes scientific', *New Scientist*, 14 August.

Strong, R. (1986) 'Sponsorship and the Arts', *The House Magazine*, 14 February.
US Department of Health and Human Services (1989), *Reducing the health consequences of smoking - 25 years of Progress*, A report of the Surgeon General, Public Health Service. Centres for Diseases Control, Centre for Chronic Disease Prevention and Health Promotion, Office of Smoking and Health. DHHS Publication no. (CDC) 89-8411.

Veitch, A. and Hencke, D. (1987), *The Guardian*, 19 February.

Watts, S. (1992), *The Independent*, 20 July.

7 Seat belts and freedom of the individual

Melvyn D. Read

On the 31 July 1991, it became compulsory for all drivers and passengers, including those travelling in the rear of motor cars to wear safety belts where fitted in the vehicle. It was the culmination of an arduous campaign by a number of Peers and Members of Parliament (MPs) and, more recently, government Ministers. The impact of the legislation in the United Kingdom, with some 16 million registered vehicles, is immense. At some time or other about 25 million people will be affected. The legislation was the last of a series of proposals designed to reduce the number of fatalities and serious injuries on the roads each year. Yet, despite these good intentions, measures to make the wearing of seat belts mandatory have faced consistent and long term opposition from within Parliament. Indeed, as I shall show, success was only made possible following the dramatic intervention of the Conservative Government and, in the latter stages, support from a Minister of Transport who was convinced of the need for compulsion.

The aim of this Chapter, then, is to examine why measures designed to save lives, face such stiff opposition. It is of interest because, unlike many of the other preventive health policies under discussion, the seat belt controversy focuses overtly on the 'freedom of the individual' as a major constraint to the adoption of prevention. I begin by considering the argument both for and against the use of seat belts, rather than the issue of compulsion. I will show that there is conflicting evidence about the effectiveness of seat restraints. On the one hand, research and the intellectual appeal suggests that the use of belts in motor vehicles saves lives. On the other, Adams and others argue cogently that the reduction in fatalities and serious injury is a function of change in driving behaviour combined with a number of exogenous effects. Secondly, I shall examine the various legislative proposals which have been introduced into the

Houses of Parliament and demonstrate how these proposals have been blocked by a group of Lords and 'cross-party' MPs united by their ideological opposition to such legislation.

In the final section I deal with the success of legislation in order to show how changing government attitudes won the day for supporters of compulsion. I indicate how the initial measure to make the use of front seat belts compulsory was a precursor of mandatory rear seat belt use as well. I shall conclude that political ideology can hinder measures designed to help the individual help themselves even where that same ideological stance underpins that preferred behavioural pattern for the individual.

The arguments for and against the use of seat belts

Although the seat belt controversy originated in the early 1960s, it did not become a part of the 'real' political agenda until government began to take a serious look at the financing of public health. The basis for concern focused on the number of people killed or injured on the road. In 1976, 6,600 people were killed and 80,800 people seriously injured (HMSO, 1977). Although these figures seem high, they compare favourably with figures for 1961 when there were 6,900 fatalities and 85,000 people seriously injured. Although the statistics suggest a small decline these should be seen in the context of a 60 per cent increase in the number of licensed vehicles between those years.

The reduction in the death toll on the road was a consequence of a number of preventive measures undertaken by a number of interested agencies: education by the police and road safety officers; safer car design; stricter control over motor vehicles (MOT); better quality roads and lighting and legislation such as the compulsory wearing of crash helmets for motor cyclists. However, since so many people are still killed or seriously injured in road traffic accidents, despite these preventive measures, part of the problem clearly lies with the behaviour of individual drivers. To reduce the toll of dead and injured further, some form of state action would be needed to force individuals to make behavioural change. It is here that the tension between the interests of the individual (to preserve their own freedom) and the public (to have safer roads) can be found. This tension has to be managed by the state.

Although drivers, and passengers, of cars are at much less risk than other categories of road user, there are many more of them. Nearly twice as many occupants of motor vehicles are killed or seriously injured than bicycle riders. In the light of this, two preventive measures, aimed particularly at vehicle drivers and front seat passengers, were given careful consideration. The first dealt with drinking (recognised as the most urgent problem) and the second would make the wearing of seat belts mandatory.

The *Road Traffic Act* of 1967 introduced the first per se law outside the Nordic countries; the three countries of Scandinavia and Finland (Ross, 1984). The Act made it an offence to drive, or attempt to drive, a vehicle on a road or other public place when drunk. Being drunk was defined as having a Blood Alcohol Concentration (BAC) in excess of 0.08 per cent. (1) A proposal to test randomly selected drivers was abandoned following vigorous political opposition (Evans, 1991, p.193). In 1983, Britain adopted a legal limit of alcohol in breath of 35 yg of alcohol per 100 ml of breath; this corresponds to 0.08 per cent BAC. (2) The effect was almost immediate; the reduction in fatalities and serious injuries was one of the largest changes associated with any intervention observed in traffic safety.

Back in 1966, almost 40 per cent of drivers aged between 20 and 40 and killed on the road had blood alcohol levels greater than 80 mgm per 100 ml. Following the introduction of the breath test the proportion of fatalities for this age group fell to 20 per cent. Overall, recorded deaths and serious injuries fell by about 12 per cent; from 30,697 in 1967 to 28,654 in 1968. Although it was estimated that about 1,000 lives would be saved in the first year official figures suggest that the number of vehicle users killed fell by just 307; from 4,355 to 4,048. However, the number of seriously injured and slightly injured vehicle users, of all ages, fell from 281,344 to 261,509; just under 20,000. By the end of 1969, two years after the introduction of the legislation, the number of vehicle users killed or injured had climbed to pre-legislation levels.

As we can see from Fig. 1, in the years following the introduction of the drink-driving legislation fatalities continued to rise. By 1972 the number of deaths annually had reached the levels of 1967 (HMSO, 1979). However, in 1972, the number of occupants killed in motor accidents began, what became, a continuous downward trend.

John Adams (1981, 1985a, 1985b) has consistently argued that the 'dramatic reductions' were a consequence of changes in road user behaviour (1985b, p. 226). He proposed that: 'The long-term decrease in death rates ... is much more plausibly attributable to myriad behavioural adjustments in response to perceived increases in the threat to traffic (1985b)'. What we can see in the official statistics, then, is the effect of the increase in petrol prices, which occurred in 1973, combined with the imposition of a speed limit of 50 mph.

Fig. 2 shows that the number of deaths per 100 million vehicle kilometres travelled was falling quite dramatically. We can explain this in terms of better roads, better vehicle construction and other safety measures which governed road user behaviour. We may argue, then, that legislative intervention had little long-term effect although it did have an immediate, short-term effect on road deaths. Adams identifies the problem as being legislation which is ahead of public opinion and therefore nullified by non-observance and non-enforcement (1985a).

As late as 1984, drink and driving offences were not considered to be a serious crime. In February of that year, prisoners who received exemplary custodial sentences for drink driving offences were released because the police had no satisfactory accommodation for them (*The Guardian*, 8 February , 1984). However, as the decade progressed a more rigourous attitude to drink driving was adopted. Between 1978 and 1990 the number of drivers breathalysed increased almost three fold; from 31,531 to 91,661 (HMSO, 1992). However, the number of positive tests (and refusals) declined from 10,543 to 8,073. This suggests that drivers have become more conscious of being caught and that they are more aware of their responsibilities when driving. In more recent years, then, the police have taken a much more active role in identifying drunk drivers and have given a much higher profile to anti-drink driving campaigns. However, the number of arrests made over the Christmas period of 1992 show that there remains a hard-core of drivers who refuse to take notice of calls for behavioural change. (3)

Fig.1 Road Accidents: Deaths 1926–1980

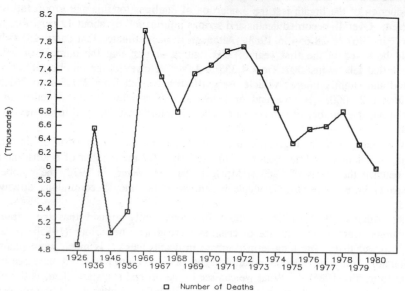

□   Number of Deaths

Fig.2 Road Accidents:Deaths 1969–1990

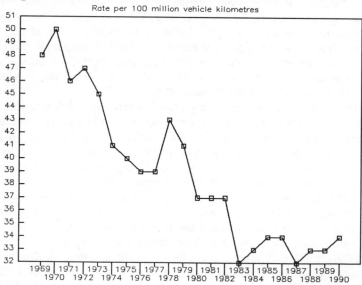

As we can see from the continuing fall in the number of deaths and serious accidents, and as John Adams has consistently argued, there must be some question about the need for seat belts. Part of the problem surrounds the difficulty associated with accurate measurement of restraint effectiveness. Evans (1991) quite rightly points out that simple comparisons should not be made. It is not enough to estimate the effectiveness of seat belts simply by comparing the percentage of fatally injured drivers, which police reports indicate were wearing the device, to the percentage of all drivers wearing seat belts, as determined by independent observation.

Other researchers argue that drivers behave differently when wearing seat belts (O'Day and Flora, 1982; O'Neill et al., 1985). Not only do they tend to be more careful but even their accidents are less severe (Campbell, 1987). The reliability of reported data has been questioned. It is possible to be fairly sure if a fatally injured driver was wearing a seat belt. It is not possible, however, to be so certain about vehicle occupants who are merely injured. Because it is an offence not to wear a seat belt admitting to this is to confess to a crime. While recognising the problem of accurate data, Evans (1986) estimated that the fatality reducing effectiveness of seat belts was 42.9 per cent (+ or - 3.8 per cent) for drivers and 39.2 per cent (+ or - 4.3 per cent) for front right-seat passengers.

Seat belts operate in two ways: they prevent ejection from the vehicle and reduce the severity with which the occupant comes into contact with the vehicle's interior. In the United Kingdom, a study showed that of 919 crashes there were just 2 cases of a belted occupant being completely ejected. The authors concluded that belt use reduces the ratio of ejection by a factor of 39 (cited in Evans, 1991, p. 232). Further evidence suggests that 25.7 per cent of unbelted drivers who were killed were thrown from the vehicle and that almost half the effectiveness of seat belts is in preventing ejection. When ejection is removed from the equation the value of seat restraints falls to just 14 per cent for drivers and 8 per cent for passengers.

If restraint is so effective then, clearly, driving can be made safer by a relatively simple change in occupant behaviour. However, as we shall see, some MPs consider this requirement to be a major philosophical issue concerning freedom of the individual and choice. In response to this argument it is possible to show that, unlike many preventive measures, this adjustment affects neither social life nor does it make excessive demands on people.

Government action

In this section I look at the various legislative attempts to introduce seat belt legislation. Legislation was passed in 1961 which required all new vehicles, built after 1 April 1965, to have seat belts fitted (HC Debates, vol. 636, col. 456, 8 March, 1961). Despite this positive move, a survey carried out by Gallup, 13 years later, showed that just 27 per cent of drivers used them (Gallup, 1976). (4) The implication was clear; if seat belts were to be used to prevent more deaths and injuries, some element of compulsion was necessary. It was not until 1974 that the issue was placed on the political agenda.

Road Traffic Bill (1973)

The first serious attempt to make the use of seat belts mandatory began in the House of Lords. (5)   Indeed, the Lords regard it as something of a tradition to initiate 'legislation on the vital subject of road traffic' (HL Debates, vol. 346, col. 819, 15 November, 1973).

It was during the Second Reading of the *Road Traffic Bill* (1973) that Lord Montague announced his intention to introduce a simple Clause giving government regulatory powers to implement the mandatory wearing of seat belts, by Statutory Instrument. Although his intention was to use a later stage, procedural opposition to the proposal was immediate. Objections were raised concerning the enforcement of the legislation and on the restrictions they would place on individual liberty (HL Debates, vol. 346, col. 861-3, 15 November, 1973).

The government accepted the amendment as necessary because the public was unwilling 'to take advice' on this issue. Although the Bill received a Second Reading (despite objections in the Commons) it failed to progress further because a General Election was called soon after and it fell.

Road Traffic Bill (1974)

In a study of road accidents the 1974 Annual Report of the Transport and Road Research Laboratory (TRRL) drew attention to the type of injuries sustained by vehicle users. Drivers suffering severe injuries generally experienced: fracture of the femur; head injuries; and chest injuries (which tended to be the most likely to cause fatality). Passengers received head injuries owing to impacting with the windscreen or the fascia panel. The findings indicated a 'considerable reduction in levels of injury amongst the belted sample' (TRRL,1974, p. 35). However, this was qualified by the small size of the sample; a reliable pattern of injury could not be established.

Encouraged by this report, the new *Road Traffic Bill* (1974) became the focus for attention for those wishing to introduce seat belt legislation. Based on the *Road Traffic Bill* (1973) from the previous Session, it was introduced into the House of Lords in May, 1974. The Lords were reminded of the Clause dealing with seat belts and the government spokesman, Lord Harris, indicated government support for a measure, which had been revised and clarified, because they are convinced that this is right' (HL Debates, vol. 351, col. 1565, 23 May, 1974).

There was active and organised resistance when the Clause was re-introduced during the Committee of the Whole House, although general support for the measure was shown when an attempt to delete the Clause was defeated by 66 votes to 55 (HL Debates, vol. 352, col. 379-382, 11 June 1974).

The proposal was subject to further opposition at Report. There were calls for the Clause to be deleted; 12 of the 19 Lords who spoke during the debate supported an amendment to that effect. Despite efforts to defend the Clause on the basis of it sometimes being necessary for the state to interfere in personal and individual choices (1974, col. 1338) the Clause was rejected, 79-72 (HL Debates, vol. 352, col. 1367-1368, 25 June 1974). A Third Reading was given on 27 June, 1974 (HL Debates, vol. 352, col. 1712, 27 June 1974).

Although government indicated support for a seat belt proposal re-introduced when the *Road Traffic Bill* went to the Commons in July 1974, owing to technical reasons the proposal was defeated. Without the Clause the *Road Traffic Bill* received Royal Assent on 31 July 1974.

Road Traffic (Seat Belts) Bill, 1974

In the following year Parliament received the first traffic Bill dealing exclusively with seat belts. Following the format of previous proposals, the Bill was designed to provide the Minister of Transport with powers to compel drivers and front seat passengers to wear seat belts. Although seemingly a decisive move the measure was, in fact, rather half-hearted. The Second Reading began at 21.00, on 21 November 1974. The debate lasted for just one hour and was then adjourned. The Minister told the House that at some future date time was to be made available for further discussion. None was forthcoming and the Bill was withdrawn. (6)

Road Traffic (Seat Belts) Bill, 1976

Following the abortive *Road Traffic (Seat Belts) Bill* (1974), Dr John Gilbert, the new Minister of Transport, re-introduced the proposal. He told the House that the basic ideas contained within the Bill had received the support of successive governments. However, it was acknowledged that it was an issue which 'touches on a question which has always, rightly (been), considered to be of the highest importance - the duty of the State with respect to the liberty of the individual' (HC Debates, vol. 878, col. 848, 1976). Support for the proposal tended to be 'cross party' while the opposition was predominantly Conservative.

During the Committee Stage there was vigorous opposition to the substance of the Bill (largely by Conservatives Ronald Bell and Norman Fowler) again on the basis that it was both a threat to individual liberty and that it could not be enforced. When the Bill was Reported back on 25 June, 1976, it was filibustered by a determined opposition.

In fact, the Bill had been put down for further debate on 14th October 1976 but too few Members were present to force a vote. (7) Despite this set back William Rodgers (Gilbert's successor) re-affirmed his support for compulsion but could see no gap in a crowded parliamentary time-table (*The Times*, 16 December, p. 27, 1976).

In the wake of this failure, pressure was brought to bear on government to make a really positive effort to legislate in favour of compulsion. At the end of 1976, the *British Medical Journal* (BMJ) called for child restraints. It was argued that cars are designed for adults rather than children and allowance had to be made for changes in the physical development of children until such time that they could wear adult seat belts. Referring to a survey carried out in 1974, the *BMJ* pointed to research which showed that when travelling in motor vehicles involved in accidents children who were protected suffered less severe injuries than unprotected children travelling in the same car (*BMJ*, 31 December 1976).

Compulsion as a preventive measure, was now full square part of the political agenda. On the 23 September 1977 it was indicated that the mandatory use of seat belts, for an experimental period only, was to be introduced into Northern Ireland. The move came following a concerted campaign of police pressure in the wake of high levels of fatalities and injuries. In 1976, 300 people had been killed in motor vehicle accidents compared to 247 killed by terrorist action.

The Minister of Transport told Northern Ireland MPs that he had consulted with groups in the Province and recognised that the majority of deaths on the roads was a consequence of drink and poor driving. But he insisted that the compulsory use of seat belts would go some way to reducing the carnage on the roads.

Despite this clear indication of intent the emphasis remained on persuasion rather than compulsion. As if to demonstrate the importance of education the Minister of Transport announced the launch of a pro-seat belts campaign which would cost £705,000 (*The Times*, 7 February, p. 4, 1978). In April the Medical Commission on Accident Prevention (8) condemned the delay in introducing compulsion. A few weeks later a national campaign aimed at persuading drivers and passengers to wear seat belts in the course of short journeys was announced. The £1,162,000 campaign was to counter 'widely held belief that belts are unnecessary for short journeys around town (*The Times*, 6 May 1978)'. In 1977, the TRRL had proposed that the 'overall benefits of wearing seat belts have been confirmed again'. The findings of the Laboratory reported a probability of being badly injured when wearing seat belts as being reduced to less than half (TRRL, 1977, p. 61). In June 1978, the TRRL reported that 6 out of 10 motorists were opposed to compulsion. Although only 39 per cent of sampled drivers supported such a measure 90 per cent thought that belts gave effective protection while nearly half wore seat restraints all the time (*The Times*, 15 June, 1978).

On 13 June 1978 William Rodgers presided over the first government conference on road safety. David Ennals, Secretary of State for Social Services, told the conference:

> I admit to being disappointed at the progress on this. The overwhelming majority of the public recognize that wearing belts is an effective way of reducing casualties (*The Times*, 14 June, 1978).

Road Traffic (Seat Belts) Bill, 1979

At the October 1978 annual conference of the Royal Society for the Prevention of Accidents (RoSPA) the issue of seat belts was raised. The issue was not clear cut and there was some dispute. Delegates refused to vote on the direct issue of compulsion, rather, they debated a motion calling for legislation to ensure road users comply with measures 'for their own safety' by a majority of two to one.

The arguments were similar to these heard in Parliament. The deputy president of the Society (Lord Nugent) argued that seat belt legislation was a 'safety measure of such fundamental value for saving life and limb that it should be backed by the law' while others saw 'compulsion hit[ting] at the very fundamentals of democracy'. Tony Lee, Director of public affairs for the RAC, indicated his support for the campaign but did not accept that the time had come for compulsion (*The Times*, 1 November 1979).

In November 1978, William Rodgers told the House of Commons, in a written reply, that wearing seat belts would become compulsory in the summer of 1979 (HC Debates, vol. 957, col. 3, 2 November, 1978) so it was no surprise when the government embarked upon a third government attempt to introduce legislation.

Of the 27 MPs who made speeches at the Second Reading (March 1979) the 13 Labour MPs were almost unanimous in their support for the Bill while the 14 Conservative Members were divided. The Opposition declared its support for seat belts but was opposed to compulsion and rejected the creation of a new criminal offence which was difficult to enforce. Attention was drawn to the relations between the police and the public and it was suggested that those relations would be soured if such an unacceptable law were to be enforced. In fact, the Magistrates' Association was also opposed to the law because they would have to operate it. The House was given a 'free vote' which the government won 244-147 (HC DEbates, vol 946, col. 1829-1832, 22 March 1979). Despite this victory the Bill was lost once more, on this occasion, owing to the 1979 General Election.

An examination of government attempts to introduce legislation to make wearing of seat belts compulsory, demonstrates the controversial nature of this 'simple' issue. Despite expressed support for the measure, the government attitude was at best ambivalent. Two points are worth noting. First, successive governments shied away from giving the support necessary for such a controversial matter to succeed. Five attempts by government to introduce legislation, failed. The use of a 'free' vote is an indication that government was wary of becoming embroiled in a controversy which might offend both MPs and a large section of the public. Secondly, it illustrates how important ideology, that is of freedom of the individual and the right to choose, can be to some members of the legislature. This is clear since such issues tend to be regarded as 'cross-party' and are frequentnly decided without the constraint of party discipline. Indeed, such is the strength of ideology that on this issue, unlike a controversial issue like AIDS, it receives an almost procedural like expression during debates in the House of Commons.

Private Members' Bills

In contrast to those members opposed to restrictions on the freedom of the individual a number of MPs at Westminster share a more collectivist approach to the trade off between public and individual interest. In the light of the support which such proposals had engendered coupled with his interest in transport, Neil Carmichael (Labour MP: Kelvingrove) used his second place in the annual private members' ballot to promote the *Road Transport (Seat Belts) Bill*. Having drawn such a high position, he was at least assured of a debate and a vote. However, his cause was not helped by John Corrie (Conservative MP: Ayrshire North and Bute) having drawn first place and introducing the even more controversial, *Abortion (Amendment) Bill*.

The Second Reading began in July, 1979 and support had been received from the police, AA, and interested individuals. Opposition to the Bill in the House of Commons was orchestrated by Ivan Lawrence and Ronald Bell and, outside the House, the RAC looked upon compulsion with disfavour.

David Mellor, making his Maiden Speech, invoked the image of 'big brotherism' (HC Debates, vol. 970, col. 2199, 20 July, 1979) but only served to underpin the objections which were already so well rehearsed. These objections included: a threat to personal liberty; the inability to enforce such legislation; the idea that seat belts were inherently dangerous; and that further powers should not be given to the executive. In reply, supporters of the Bill argued that not only was this the correct way to reduce death and serious injury on the roads but that the threat to personal freedom was more imagined than real.

Concern about the executive powers to be given to government was carried over into the Committee Stage. Throughout the five days spent in Committee fears were raised about giving the Minister of Transport too much power but finally the Bill was allowed out of Committee. This was in part a strategic move enabling opponents to continue their campaign at Report stage, which took place on 22 February, 1980.

The amount of time at Report was unusually generous. On the first day a new Clause was introduced into the Bill which required the Minister to report on the operation of the Act within two years and then annually. However, opponents were able to 'talk-out' the Bill.

On the second day at Report, 7 March 1980, discussion continued about the new Clause. Fears were once again expressed about the bureaucracy which would emanate from this 'unnecessary' legislation and the need to monitor the Act. The Bill was 'talked-out' once more. A call for a closure motion was passed 45-12 (HC Debates, vol. 981, col. 883-4, 7 March 1980). However, Standing Order 13 (Majority for Closure) prescribed that at least 100 supporters of the motion should be present. Although the Bill was set down to continue on another day, there was insufficient Parliamentary time during remainder of the Session so the Bill fell yet again.

Success for seat belt legislation

It was now some fifteen years since it had become compulsory for seat belts to be fitted into motor vehicles. Yet the introduction for their mandatory use seemed a long way off. Indeed, with the election of a Conservative government, which stressed the importance of the freedom of the individual, compulsion seemed unlikely. Yet, despite these seemingly insurmountable obstacles success was just around the corner. This section examines the successful negotiation of the Bill through the House of Commons.

In June 1980 Patrick Jenkin, Secretary of State for the Social Services, told the Spinal Injuries Association that compulsion was inevitable (*The Times*, 12 June, 1980). In July, the British Medical Association's (BMA's) Annual Representative meeting at Newcastle, passed a motion calling for the compulsory wearing of seat belts (*The Times*, 9 July 1980). In October, government launched three safety campaigns; drinking and driving, cyclists, and seat belts. This was followed in November by a call from Dr. J. Havard at the BMA Conference on Road Accidents, to support the new Bill to be introduced into the House of Lords. Havard had written to all members of the Lords urging them to vote for the Bill. He argued that more education on road safety was needed, particularly for the young. In fact, he suggested that this matter should be given at least as much time in schools as sex education (*The Times*, 24 November 1980).

Safety of Children in Cars Bill

The campaign to introduce compulsion re-opened when Labour MP Barry Sheerman drew 7th place in the annual Ballot. He chose to introduce a road safety measure; *Safety of Children in Cars Bill*. This was related to previous Bills but dealt with children in cars rather than adults. The First Reading took place on 14 January 1981, but was soon withdrawn to allow the government to incorporate the provisions of the Bill into their own Transport Bill.

In the meantime, the *Road Traffic (Seat Belts) Bill* was reintroduced into the Lords with Lord Nugent arguing, once again, that the seat belt proposal was not a limitation of liberty to which serious objection could be made. Even though Lord Balfour argued that studies from other countries showed that the reduction in injuries also corresponded to the introduction of other road safety measures, his Amendment was defeated (HL Debates, vol. 415, col. 960, 11 November, 1980). With the defeat of Balfour's amendment the Bill received its Second Reading but failed to progress further because of the 'well known vulnerability of Private Members' Bill to any opposition in the House of Commons' (HL Debates, vol. 421, col. 323, 11 June, 1981).

Meanwhile, during the Standing Committee of the government's *Transport Bill* (1981), Barry Sheerman introduced the Clause which required all children under 13 years of age to wear restraints if a front seat passenger. As we saw above, this proposal had government support. Supporters of general compulsion were concerned about the inclusion of this measure since it made their task more difficult particularly since the government intended to use a guillotine timetable, at all stages of the Bill, which would limit discussion on the wider aspects of the seat belts issue. An attempt was made to introduce a new Clause into the Bill which would have made compulsion general, but this idea was rejected by the Speaker.

However, general compulsion was still on the agenda in the Lords. The government's view was that the 'duty to care for children who are not old enough to look after their own safety override factors which must be considered in relation to the compulsory wearing of seat belts by adults' (HL Debates, vol. 421, col. 326, 11 June, 1981). Lord Nugent introduced an amendment to provide the Secretary of State for Transport with enabling powers to make regulations covering the compulsory use of seat belts. Importantly, it was made known that the government accepted the proposition that seat belts saved lives and substantially reduced the risk of serious injury so it appeared as though the technical debate over the usefulness of seat belts had been resolved.

In addition, there was now 'much support for the new Clause from a variety of quarters'. Even the RAC was stressing the importance of the maximum voluntary use of restraint harnesses. The overwhelming majority of very respected organizations favoured compulsion because it was the most effective means of achieving greater use (HL Debates, vol. 421, col. 357-359, 11 June, 1981).

At Third Reading two amendments were agreed. First, each person was made responsible for wearing his/her own seat belt. Second, a three month period was made available for consultation with interested parties. This would be followed by a three year period after which an initial report on the operation of the Act would be prepared.

On returning to the Commons, to discuss the Lords' amendments, the Bill was still subject to the guillotine and there was still opposition which revolved around 'the existing right to wear or not to wear a seat belt as the individual thought fit'. But, Norman Fowler, now Secretary of State for Transport, stressed that this measure was not a party matter. The issue was not about wearing seat belts but, rather, about compulsion because failure to comply would become a criminal offence. A vote took place on a motion to reject the Lord's amendment but it was defeated. The *Transport Bill*, which included a provision for the mandatory use of seat belts, was enacted.

Under the *Transport Bill*, the Minister of Transport was given powers to make regulations requiring drivers and front seat passengers to wear seat belts. After 7 months of negotiations with interested parties, draft regulations were presented in July, 1982. Nine days later, Lynda Chalker, Under Secretary of State for Transport, asked the House to approve the regulations. Despite somewhat muted opposition, the Regulations were approved by the House of Commons and subsequently by the Lords as well.

The Regulations came into operation on 31 January, 1983. Three years later they were confirmed with the approval of the *Motor Vehicle (Wearing Seat Belts) Regulation, 1982*.

Compulsory use of rear seat belts

Belt use was closely monitored before and after the law came into effect, at 55 Department of Transport traffic census sites throughout Britain. They reported a large increase in the use of seat belts to comply with the law. Usage rose from 40 per cent before the law to about 90 per cent after it came into operation. Quite clearly, then, the United Kingdom with over 16 million cars had the largest population affected by a single law.

Scott and Willis (1985) conclude that there was approximately a 20 per cent reduction in fatal and serious casualties to car drivers and van occupants. For front seat passengers the reduction was 30 per cent. Broughton (1988), in examining long-term trends in total British fatalities for unit distance of travel, estimated a 17 per cent reduction in fatalities and serious injuries.

A further study was undertaken by Rutherford, Greenfield, Hayes and Nelson, who examined 15 hospitals; 8 in England, 4 in Northern Ireland, 2 in Scotland and 1 in Wales. They compared the number of people requiring hospital attention, following motor vehicle accidents, in the year before and the year following the implementation of the legislation. The study showed: a 15 per cent reduction in the number of patients brought into hospital; a 25 per cent reduction in those requiring admission to a ward; and a similar fall in those needing to occupy a bed. However, the research detected an apparent increase in the number of injuries to the sturnum and in the incidents of sprained necks. The authors conclude that one consequence of the use of seat belts was a degree of injury substitution.

In February 1986, the Department of Transport published a report which estimated that between 200 and 400 lives were saved each year owing to seat belts. Two studies carried out by the TRRL, highlighted the benefits gained from the use of child restraints. The first report provided evidence that such restraints reduced the overall risk of injury by two-thirds. The second, published in May 1987, suggested that the risk for children, under four years of age, was reduced by three-quarters. As a consequence, the Department of Transport encouraged both the fitting, and use, of rear restraints for both children and adults.

Unlike previous Transport Ministers, Peter Bottomley was committed to the use of child restraints in motor vehicles. So, when Stephen Day introduced his private members' bill, *Motor Vehicles (Wearing of Seat Belts by Children)* (1988) he could rely on government support. The Bill required that children under the age of 14 should be restrained by seat belts in the rear seats of cars where fitted. In 1986, 89 per cent of child car occupant casualties were seated in the rear, while 91 per cent of child fatalities were among those in the rear of vehicles. The successful Clause in the *Transport Act* (1981) had covered children in front seats only. The Bill had been assisted by the Parliamentary Advisory Council for Transport Safety (PACTS) together with a number of outside organizations. These included a number of police associations, accident prevention agencies, and medical groups.

Surprisingly, there was opposition along lines which by now were very familiar - the measures would not have the desired effect (Gary Waller); that the House legislated in too many areas of human behaviour (Eric Forth); that there was too much legislation which interfered with personal responsibility (Teresa Gorman) (HC Debates, vol. 126, cols. 1281-1288, 5 February; vol. 133, cols. 619 and 646, 13 May, 1988). This was not enough to stop the Bill.

By the time of the Third Reading the government were asked in the Lords why its views on compulsion had changed since 1981. The reply was that:

> Times have changed. Compulsory seat-belt wearing has come into force since that time. And it has proved to be very popular. ... use went up almost overnight ... to 95 per cent. It has remained at that level (HL Debates, vol. 498, col. 1209, 27 June, 1988).

The Bill completed its passage through Westminster in 21 June 1988 and received the Royal Assent on 28 June 1988 (HC Debates, vol. 136, col. 219, 28 June 1988). On the following day Paul Channon announced his intention to consult with interested parties before the Act was brought into force.

Road Traffic Bill (1988)

This Bill consolidated the *Criminal Justice Bill* and the *Motor Vehicle (Wearing of Seat Belts by Children) Bill* neither of which had been enacted. It was referred to the Joint Committee on Consolidation Bills and was discharged without amendment (HL Debates, vol. 498, col. 832, 20 June, 1988). The Third Reading was passed without debate. The importance of the Bill would be seen two years later when the Transport Minister was able to use the provisions of the Act to make the use of rear seat belts compulsory for adults.

Indeed, it was not long before the idea of compulsory rear seat restraints for adults reached the political agenda. Peter Bottomley gave support to a draft European Community directive calling for seat belts to be used in mini-buses. Announcing this measure, the Minister stated that: 'The Department is advising drivers that ... seat belts should be worn by rear seat passengers ... wherever possible' (HC Debates, vol. 145, col. 192, 18 January, 1989). Government support was underscored when Robert Atkins, Minister of State for Transport, launched the nationwide campaign to *Belt Up in the Back*. Dr Murray Mackay, Vice-Chairman of PACTS, said that the next step should be to make rear seat belts compulsory for all.   It was emphasized that no Government plans to implement such a measure existed.

By 1990, pressure for general compulsion was mounting.   On 28 March 1990, it was suggested that the use of rear seat belts might become obligatory for all passengers and drivers.   The point at which compulsion would be possible was when 70 per cent of motor vehicles were fitted with rear seat belts.   Evidence from the TRRL indicated that since legislation had been passed, 80 per cent of children were wearing restraints. This was followed, in April 1990, by a survey published by PACTS which argued that rear seat belts would reduce fatal accidents and serious injury by two-thirds.   Stephen Day, co-chair of PACTS, launched a campaign to make people more aware of the need for rear seat belts.

On 3 June 1990, the ideological argument against compulsion received a massive blow.   In a major coach accident at Auxerre, France, 11 people were killed and 18 persons injured.   In response, the Department of Transport (DoT) was motivated to make the use of seat belts compulsory in all public service vehicles.   Five days later, the Secretary of State for Transport met the representatives of the Bus and Coach Council to discuss the fitting of seat belts in these vehicles.   In fact, the issue of seat belts on coaches had been raised fourteen years previously.   In 1977, the TRRL reported that, 'the proposed standard for dynamic and static tests to ensure that coach seat occupants are restrained in place during frontal impacts has been agreed between the DoT, the Society of Motor Manufacturers and Traders and the Laboratory' (TRRL,1977:62).

The outcome was that the Council undertook to recommend to its members that all new vehicles purchased should have seat belts fitted.   Following this meeting, Departmental officials met the representatives again in July, to discuss the fitting of restraints in existing vehicles.

On 18 July 1990, Peter Atkins announced:

> Now that the majority of cars have rear seat belts fitted, the
> time is approaching when it would be reasonable to consider the
> introduction of mandatory wearing by adults (HC Debates, vol.
> 176 , col. 587, 18 July, 1990).

By November, government support for compulsion was total.   Christopher Chope, Minister for Road and Transport, summed up the reasons for this change of heart.   Of rear seat belts, he stated:

> I consider (them) to be the single most important measure
> which can be taken by the Government further to reduce deaths
> and injuries to car occupants ... I am issuing a consultation
> paper this morning inviting comments on a proposal to extend
> the law on seat belt wearing ... to apply to adults as well as
> children in rear seats of vehicles where seat belts are fitted (HC
> Debates, vol. 180, col. 808, 16 November 1990).

It was, he continued, a shared responsibility:

> A feature of the past two or three years has been the

development of an alliance of interests, involving the public
and private sector. Reflecting this growing concern, and to
some degree fostering it, is the responsible attitude of the media
which ... campaigns for change (HC Debates, vol. 180, col.
809, 16 November, 1990).

Despite the fact that in earlier years the public had not responded positively to
exhortations to wear seat belts there was a discernible change in attitude. The
acceptance of seat belts, and the increased incidence of wearing them, was seen as a
feature of the positive media coverage which underpinned public willingness to use
restraints. Evans (1991), argues that the media was successful because it was modest
and unobtrusive and did not involve enforcement. Shinar and McKnight (1985) had
previously found similar examples of public information increasing compliance with
traffic laws. They argue that 'public information has been widely used to encourage
compliance with both traffic laws and safe driving practice'. However, there must
also be an increase in enforcement of the relevant legislation. In this case, most of the
information drivers were receiving concerned the efforts that were being made to
enforce existing regulations. This suggests that those regulations have to be in place
for the enforcement and the information to have its full effect. This view contradicts
that held by Adams that legislation will be nullified if it is in advance of public opinion
(see above).

Indeed, support for the introduction of compulsion to wear seat belts was coming
from a great diversity of interests. The National Licensed Victuallers Association had
promoted the use of low-alcohol beers in order to reduce the number of drink related
accidents. However, it also formed part of a road safety promotion organized by the
DoT. Kwik-Fit, Autoglass and Halfords sponsored these initiatives while general
support came from the motoring organizations, AA and RAC, and the police.

The Government used the period to 31 January 1991, as an opportunity to consult
with interested parties. Backing came from PACTS, RoSPA, the police, motoring
organizations and local authorities. With this support and the changing attitude to
mandatory use of seat belts, the Minister was able to use the regulations provided by
the Road Traffic Act (1988). On the 31 July 1991, it became compulsory for all
motor vehicle passengers to use rear seat belts, where fitted.

Conclusion

Despite the focus of attention on preventive health policies, successive Governments
have maintained an almost ambivalent attitude to the compulsory wearing of seat belts.
That being said, once committed to compulsion regulations were quickly implemented.
However, it remains clear that the accepted ideological stance of the Conservative
government would be opposed to forcing such restrictions upon individuals even where
that restriction is meant to improve the lot of individuals.

What seems clear, however, is that Westminster provides a forum where ideological
preferences are most obvious. It is in the Chambers that an almost physical expression
of these preferences will manifest themselves. Yet, there is a contradiction between
'individualists' who promote freedom and individual responsibility and the
'collectivists' who expound the notion of 'public good' and see a role for the state in

the affairs of the citizen.

Given that all governments have tended to hesitate in this area, it is not surprising that Conservative members also adopt an anti-paternalistic, anti-nanny state approach to seat belts. For some MPs, then, freedom of the individual remains a higher priority than protecting the individual from harm. In this sense ideology actually hinders particular preventive measures even where that same ideology supports proposals under which such measures become necessary. There is, then, a conflict between freedom of an individual and the cost incurred when that individual is killed or seriously injured. Thus, for individualists, there is a clear contradiction between freedom and health.

Perhaps the most crucial feature of this contradiction, however, is that such ideology rarely can be maintained in the face of strong evidence which seemingly calls it into question. When it becomes clear to government that it is sensible to impose regulations for both financial and social reasons the ideological position is lost. So, despite the strong feelings which had initially opposed the introduction of compulsory seat belts for drivers and front seat passengers it was possible to pass measures which went well beyond the proposals as envisaged, and defended, during the 1970s and early 1980s.

Footnotes

1) Blood Alcohol Concentration (BAC) is the per cent, by weight, of alcohol in the blood.

2) A breath measurement of g/L is converted to BAC in per cent by multiplying by a factor in the range of 210 to 230.

3) There seems to be a hard core of drivers who are prepared to take a risk. Following the anti-drink driving campaign undertaken at Christmas 1992, senior police officers called for random testing. The 'shocking' video had had little impact. Between 19th December and Ist January there were 300 arrests per day. The number of fatal road accidents rose by almost 6 per cent.

Although the number of positive breath tests had fallen from 4,921 in 1991 to 4,248 in 1992 this has been matched by a compensating fall in the number of tests carried out; 59,069 compared with 64,118 (*The Guardian*, 1992, 4 January).

4) The study showed that 39 per cent of drivers used them for motor way driving. A year later Gallup reported a slight increase amongst drivers who wore seat belts all the time (29 per cent) although the proportion of drivers wearing them some of the time had fallen (36 per cent).

Six months later, in March 1976, the proportion of drivers wearing seat belts all of the time had fallen again (27 per cent) although those who wore them some of the time had increased (42 per cent). Only 31 per cent of drivers reported never wearing seat restraints (Gallup, 1976). To over come this reluctance the government embarked on an expensive advertising campaign. Yet, by 1978 the Secretary of State for Transport told the House of Commons that just 31 per cent of drivers wore belts. In March

1978, another advertising campaign costing some £700,000 was launched but had little effect.

5) In fact the House of Commons had rarely given transport priority. Of the five government Bills which dealt with compulsion between 1973 and 1979, two began in the Lords and three in the Commons. Each of the five proposals petered out reflecting, perhaps, the low priority afforded to this issue. Members were allowed a free vote but Ministers did not provide the requisite support such measures require. Even though they were government Bills none passed despite the executive's dominance over the legislature in British politics (Marsh and Read, 1988, p. 157).

6) In that year 73 government Bills were enacted. *The Road Traffic (Seat Belts) Bill* was one of five Bills which was withdrawn. The other four were fairly large and complicated measures, for instance, one dealt with the Channel Tunnel.

7) A Closure motion requires at least 100 members to vote in favour of a motion which brings debate to an end and permits a vote on the Bill to take place. Without this number present the debate will continue and the proposal will be talked out.

8) The MCAP is an independent medical advisory body consisting of representatives of the 11 Royal Colleges and faculties of medicine, The British Medical Association, and 14 specialist associations.

Bibliography/references

Broughton, J. (1984), 'Predictive models of road accident fatalities', *Traffic Engineering and Control*, vol.29, pp. 296-300.

Campbell, B.J. (1987), 'Safety belt injury reduction to crash severity and front seated position', *Journal of Trauma*, vol.27, pp. 733-9.

Evans, L. (1986), 'The effectiveness of safety belts in preventing fatalities', *Accident Analysis in Prevention*, vol.18, pp. 229-41.

Evans, L. (1991), *Traffic Safety and the Driver*, Van Nostrand Reinhold, New York.

Evans, L and Schwing, R.C. (eds) (1985), *Human Behaviour and Traffic Safety*, Plenum Press, London.

Gallup Political Index (1976), Report no.189, April.

Marsh, D. and Read, M. (1988), *Private Members' Bills*, Cambridge University Press, Cambridge.

O'Day, J. and Flora, J. (1982), 'Alternative measures of restraint system effectiveness: interaction with crash severity factors', SAE paper 820798, Warrendale, P.A., Society of Automation Engineers.

Ross, H.L. (1984), *Deterring the Drinking Driver*, Lexington Books, Lexington, M.A.

Rutherford, W.H., Greenfield, T., Hayes, H.R.M. and Nelson, J.K. (1985), 'The medical effects of seat belt legislation in the United Kingdom', Office of the Chief Scientist, Research Report no.13, Department of Health and Social

Security, London.

Scott, P.P. and Willis, P.A. (1985), 'Road casualties in Great Britain the first year with seat belt legislation', Transport and Road Research Laboratory, Report no. 9, Crowthorne, Berks,

Shinar, D. and McKnight, A.J. (1985) 'Then effects of enforcement and public information', in, Evans, L. and Schwing, R.C. (eds), *Human Behaviour and Traffic Safety*, Plenum Press, London.

Transport and Road Research Laboratory (TRRL) (1974), *1974 Annual Report of the Transport and Road Research Laboratory*, Department of the Environment, HMSO, London.

Transport and Road Research Laboratory(TRRL) (1977), *1977 Annual Report of the Transport and Road Research Laboratory*, Department of the Environment, HMSO, London.

8 Purity and danger: The politicisation of drinking water quality in the eighties

Hugh Ward

In this chapter I explain why issues surrounding water quality and public health became so heavily politicised in the 1980s. The puzzle is that these issues appeared to be of greater public concern than problems which are arguably of greater significance to public health, such as smoking and lung cancer, diet and heart disease, private motoring and road deaths, or health and safety at work. To be sure, drinking water quality generated major public health problems in Britain up until the reforms of the nineteenth century and it remains a major health problem in many countries in the South. But Britain came to pride itself on the quality of its drinking water and sewage disposal as compared to the 'unsafe' arrangements in some continental countries. Although water-related legislation continued to be passed after the Public Health Acts of the nineteenth century, the most important being the *Water Act* of 1973 setting up 10 new publicly owned regional water authorities, issues surrounding drinking water quality were technical and hardly central to the political agenda. The addition of fluoride to the drinking water supply did occasion some public debate in the 1970s but the reason for this was that some saw this as a form of compulsory adulteration. Also, related issues, such as the environmental quality of British rivers, were of some concern in the post-war period. But in the light of the fact that the public health issue had been largely dormant, its re-emergence in the 1980s merits explanation.

I will argue below that no single factor can be isolated explaining the politicisation of issues surrounding water quality. Rather a number of factors combined together. The health risks that came to be of public concern arise as a result of contamination of drinking water by numerically tiny amounts of industrial, agricultural and other pollutants which are also of broader environmental concern. Despite the fact that for much of the Thatcherite 1980s the political climate was hostile for the environmental movement, as part of their new campaigning thrust, environmentalists drew increasing attention both to broad environmental issues surrounding water and to the public health issues (Ward et al., 1990). Environmental concern reciprocally fed health concerns in a way which did not occur with other preventive health issues. For a series of reasons the 1980s were a propitious time to open up the water agenda: environmental standards of rivers and groundwater declined; the environmental movement found an important political ally in the European Community (EC) which, as part of a broader move to concern itself with the environment, had attempted to control water quality; the government's moves to privatise the water industry fed public concern because of fears that the insertion of the profit motive into the industry would squeeze out investment in water quality; the privatisation debate was a unique opportunity to get the issues publicly discussed. Again, such opportunities were lacking in relation to other preventive health issues. Water has long been a symbol of purity in most cultures; and its commodification by those who attempt to sell it like any other industrial product, as the privatised water industry does, is widely seen as a danger to its symbolic status (Illich, 1985). Beside this, the health dangers some associate with drinking water include cancers and threats to the development of children, both of which have high symbolic load. The combination of the symbolisms of purity and danger here gave environmentalists resources absent in relation to other preventive health problems.

In the first section of this chapter I briefly summarise what the main public health concerns have been in the 1980s. In the second section, I follow the politics of the water industry through the 1980s, focussing first on the effects of Thatcherism on the politics of environmental regulation then on the privatisation debate. As I show in the first section, many scientists believe that water purity is not a significant public health issue in Britain. In the light of this, some may view the massive investments in clean-up which will probably occur over the next twenty years as an irrational move. In the conclusion I examine these sorts of argument in more detail. While it is true that the environmental movement was able to manipulate the symbolism of purity and danger in a way that made health risks which looked minuscule to some scientists unacceptable to many of the public, I argue that we are not making irrational investments here. However, I suggest that one scenario is that the public will become more loth to pay for clean-up as time goes by.

The scientific debate on water quality and health

Concern has been expressed about the effects upon health of a large number of things which are sometimes present in drinking water. Firstly, there are 'unusual' pollution incidents. For example contamination of drinking water by bacteria may occur, due to breakdown of chlorination plant, broken or leaking sewers, and so on. Again, there are incidents such as the dumping of the water treatment chemical aluminium sulphate into the wrong tank at the Lowermoor works in Cornwall in 1988, leading to pollution of local water supplies in the Camelford area (Cook, 1990, pp. 59-63). I have chosen not to concentrate on such incidents. Although they may cause significant adverse media and public reaction, they are probably less significant in health terms than the long-term effects of routine contamination. There is a formidable list of possible contaminants of water supplies: aluminium, which some believe to be linked to

Alzheimer's disease; heavy metal pollution, including cadmium, mercury and lead; pollution due to agrichemicals, particularly nitrates and pesticides; and other forms of industrial pollution, including those due to organic chemicals such as chlorinated solvents. Rather than attempt to cover all the issues, I will concentrate in some detail on nitrates, pesticides, and lead. The justification is that these three pollutants were arguably more important to the public debate in the 1980s. At the same time, I can illustrate most of the important themes by reference to them.

Nitrates

As I will show below, the issue of nitrate levels in drinking water was central to the politicisation of water quality in the 1980s. In fact, water is not the largest source of nitrates in the diet: most people ingest more nitrates from food than from water (Dudley, 1990, p. 19). Even at the World Health Organisation (WHO) recommended limit, the proportion of nitrates in diet coming from water has been calculated at around 55 per cent for a typical British diet (OECD, 1986, p. 53), and the recommended limit exceeds levels found in most British drinking water. Many vegetables contain inorganic nitrogen and concentrations can be increased by the use of artificial fertilisers. Also, nitrates added to foods and meat products as a preservative and to improve the appearance account for about 9 per cent of nitrate intake (Dudley, 1990, p. 24).

Nitrates, themselves, are not thought to be a significant health risk at typical dose levels. Rather, the significant risks are associated with the reduced form of nitrates, the nitrites and their reaction products. Reduction of nitrates to nitrites is usually the result of microbial action either in stored food or in the human body, most significantly in the mouth, but also in the stomach. Because of the physiology of the newborn, in bottle fed babies high levels of nitrate in drinking water which give rise to nitrites in the body may be associated with 'blue baby syndrome'. Most cases seem to be associated with levels of nitrate of 90 milligrams per litre in the water used to mix feeds - well above the WHO recommended limit (OECD, 1986, p. 51). There have only been 14 recorded cases in Britain since 1945, the last occurring in 1972. The last fatality in Britain occurring in 1950 (Dudley, 1990, p. 44).

The second set of health problems are associated with complex reactions of nitrites with amines and amides to form nitrosamines and nitrosamides (N-nitroso compounds). Many experts now believe that this can happen in the human body as well as in cooking (Dudley, 1990, p. 46). Experimental studies on animals have established that N-nitroso compounds are highly carcinogenic. The suggestion is that they may also be associated with human cancers, especially stomach cancers. However, the epidemiological studies carried out so far vary in their results, and it has been difficult to establish a causal link at concentrations currently occurring in our water (Dudley, 1990, pp. 46-47). Moreover, drinking water, and diet in general, are not the only environmental sources of these compounds, and the effects of dietary sources are difficult to separate from those of other sources, including smoking.

In 1985 the government Chief Scientist said that:

> Although a theoretical risk of a relationship between nitrate and
> cancers remains, the epidemiological evidence, looked at as a

whole, gives no support to the suggestion that nitrate is a cause of cancer in the stomach, or any other organ, in the United Kingdom (Dudley, 1990, p. 42).

Nevertheless, because of the possible established link with blue baby syndrome and the known carcinogenic properties of N-nitroso compounds, in 1971 the WHO set a recommended limit for nitrates in European drinking water at 50 milligrams per litre and a maximum acceptable limit of 100 milligrams per litre. These limits took into account other sources of nitrates and were, to some extent, precautionary. The EC Drinking Water Directive, first put forward in 1980 and effective from 1985, made 50 milligrams per litre the maximum admissible concentration, with a guide level of 25 milligrams per litre (OECD, 1986, p. 53).

Although there are a number of sources of nitrates in water, including sewage emissions, the most important source of nitrates is, in fact, agriculture (Dudley, 1990, p. 15). Use of nitrate fertilisers tripled from 1960 to 1980, and increased at from 4 to 5 per cent per annum in the 1980s. Their use was critical to the intensification of agricultural production in the post-war period, the Common Agricultural Policy (CAP) generating very strong financial incentives for use, both on cereal crops and, increasingly, on 'improved' pasture for cattle. Particularly in cereal growing areas in the east of England, nitrates run off into rivers from which drinking water is abstracted. In the long term nitrates also seep into aquifers from which drinking water is abstracted through boreholes - a problem which will continue to get worse even if measures to control nitrate use are taken now (Dudley, 1990, pp. 30-3). Nitrate pollution problems are concentrated in the areas of three water undertakings, Severn-Trent, Anglian and Thames, although Southern, Wessex and Yorkshire also have some problems. This distribution mirrors the regional distribution of intensive cereal production. However, intensification of livestock farming may cause pollution of rivers by runoffs from animal slurry and silage clamps, which are orders of magnitude more polluting than untreated sewage (Environment Select Committee, 1987, p. xxvii). The pollutants concerned include nitrates. This is a particularly significant problem in the west of England, and some argue that drinking water quality is threatened there, too (Cook, 1989, pp. 29-32).

Pesticides

Since their development in the 1940s the consumption of organic pesticides has grown very rapidly, a twenty-fold increase in world production occurring over the last 40 years (Agriculture Select Committee, 1987, p. xi). Just like nitrates, pesticides have become central to high-input-high-output agriculture, and are also widely used by local authorities and organisations like British Rail. One indicator of their importance is that the Ministry of Agriculture, Fisheries and Food (MAFF) surveys carried out between 1977 and 1981 showed that over 90 per cent of most crops were treated with pesticides (OECD, 1986, p. 131).

The harmful effects of pesticides on the environment, especially on fish and birds of prey, became central to the mobilisation of the environmental movement in the 1960s, largely through the influence of Rachel Carson's book *Silent Spring*. The organochlorines such as DDT and aldrin are of particular concern because of their high toxicity to aquatic life, their persistence in the environment, and their tendency to accumulate in the bodies of birds and animals higher up the food chain (Ellis, 1990, pp. 102-5). The environmental hazards associated with the organochlorines led to tougher mechanisms for testing and control being adopted in most countries, the phasing out of some pesticides, including DDT and aldrin, and attempts by the chemical industry to develop safer alternatives (Ellis, 1990, chapt. 9).

Our concern here is with the health effects of chronic exposure to low concentrations of pesticides in drinking water. The chronic health effects may include increased risk of some cancers, genetic mutation and, hence, birth defects and miscarriages, various forms of allergic reaction, and neurological problems. However, such effects are very difficult to pin down. One problem is that at low dose levels the latency period may be considerable. Another problem is that the breakdown products of pesticides and manufacturing impurities may be more dangerous than the original pesticide and little is known about these. Pesticides may not be the single causal factor involved, interaction effects with other carcinogens occurring. Finally, there is the problem of inadequate and incomplete data on dose levels. In the light of these problems, evidence from epidemiological studies tends to be ambiguous, although some studies do suggest that significant health risks exist (Agriculture Select Committee, 1987, pp. xiii-xiv). As a consequence, great reliance has been placed upon studies using laboratory animals when licensing new pesticides and setting permissible human dose levels. Such studies demonstrate that some pesticides are dangerous at high dose levels. This fuels the concern of environmentalists. However, the chemical industry claims that licensing procedures ensure that, given proper use, chronic effects will not occur.

Pesticides enter drinking water as a result of run off into water courses and ground waters from which drinking water is abstracted. Run off can result from routine application, accidental spillage and deliberate disposal in violation of regulations. A considerable number of common pesticides have been detected in both surface and underground water sources since rather patchy monitoring started in the early 1970s (Agriculture Select Committee, 1987, pp. xxvii). However, the government has tended to downplay the chronic health problems associated with pesticides in water:

> the concentrations being detected routinely are lower in almost all cases by several orders of magnitude than any which are likely to cause adverse effects on health (Agriculture Select Committee, 1987, p. xxvii).

In contrast, the problem of pesticides in drinking water has been taken extremely seriously in other countries, including the US, where extensive and expensive measures have been taken tightly to control pesticide levels in drinking water (Douglas and Wildavsky, 1983, chapt. 3; Rosenbaum, 1991, chapt. 6). As we shall see below, environmental groups were able to make considerable play of the fact that water samples often contain levels of pesticide higher than the maximum permissible concentrations of 0.1 g/l for each pesticide stipulated in the 1985 EC drinking water directive.

Lead

There is no controversy over the fact that 'large' doses of lead are toxic. However, far greater controversy has been occasioned by the claim that some effects observable at 'large' doses may also be present, albeit in an attenuated way, at 'moderate', and even 'low' dose levels. Particular concern has been expressed over the possible effects of 'moderate' and 'low' doses of lead on children: poorer performance in IQ tests; hyperactivity; and other behavioural abnormalities (e.g. DHSS, 1980, chapt. 7; Landsdowne and Yule, 1986, pp. 235-70). While accepting that clinical effects are established for blood lead levels greater than 80 micrograms per decilitre, the Lawther Report, commissioned by the DHSS in the late seventies, concluded: that there was no convincing evidence of deleterious effects on children at blood level concentrations below a threshold of 35 micrograms per decilitre; that there was doubt about the possible occurrence of effects in the 35-80 microgram per decilitre band (DHSS, 1980, pp. 86-8). However, since the publication of the Lawther Report experts have started to express greater concern. For instance, in their editorial conclusion to a volume on the lead debate, William Yule and Richard Landsdowne, who had earlier participated in the DHSS working party leading to the Lawther Report, conclude that: 'there is a growing body of evidence that low levels of lead exposure do have effects on children's development' (Landsdowne and Yule, 1986, p. 274), with possible losses of around five or six IQ points (Landsdowne and Yule, 1986, p. 258). Moreover, they raise doubts about the idea that there is a threshold below which effects will not be observed (Landsdowne and Yule, 1986, pp. 273-4).

Public concern in the 1980s largely centred on lead in petrol. Strong pressure from the petrochemical industries and the car industry, often articulated through the Department of Transport (DoT), led the government to stall on the lead question, while environmental groups - especially the Campaign for Lead Free Air (CLEAR) - were highly critical of the government's position and the Lawther Report on which it was based (Price, 1986; Wilson, 1983). The view expressed by the government's Chief Medical Officer in a letter to *The Times* in February 1982 that 'lead in petrol is permanently affecting the IQ of many of our children' (Wilson, 1983, p. 31) fed public concern and gave environmentalists an easy propaganda victory. Ably lead by Des Wilson, former chairman of Shelter, CLEAR was certainly a significant factor in the government's decision to give tax incentives to lead-free petrol in the 1988 and 1989 budgets, although the government's change of heart was also linked to EC pressure to make catalytic converters compulsory on many new cars (McCormick, 1991, pp. 136-40).

Although the debate centred on airborne residues from lead in petrol, concern spilled over into the question of lead in drinking water. Ingestion of lead in drinking water and from water used to cook food can be a significant contributor to overall lead intake (Moore, 1986, p. 179), especially in areas where the water supply is soft and acidic and, thus, particularly prone to dissolve lead plumbing (Moore, 1986, pp. 147-57). The problem has been particularly important in Scotland, both because of the type of water and because of the use of lead piping and lead-lined water tanks, especially in older buildings in cities. A survey carried out by the Department of the Environment (DoE) in 1975/76 found that 34.4 per cent of households in Scotland exceeded the EC standard for lead in drinking water (DoE, 1977). The ninth report of the Royal Commission on Environmental Pollution (1983) called for greater government action and the 1985 EC drinking water directive introduced a maximum acceptable concentration of 50 micrograms per litre. As we will see below, the failure of some water supplies to meet this limit once again allowed environmental groups to make political capital in the privatisation debate.

Overview

As I have shown, the general pattern has been one in which there is a high degree of uncertainty and ambiguity over long term health effects, leading to scientific controversy. The DHSS, backed by other parts of Whitehall - notably MAFF and the DoT - generally took the view that health problems are not significant at typical British dose levels. In contrast environmentalists, making use of counter-expertise, claimed that significant risks were being taken with the nation's health, backing their arguments with the failure of the British government to comply with legally binding EC directives on Member States. Although objectivity may be an aspiration of scientists and scientific institutions may function to a degree to encourage it, it is highly unlikely in the light of our current knowledge of the sociology of science that expert opinions of either government scientists or their counterparts advising environmental group are totally disengaged from their values or from their institutional affiliations (e.g. Fischhoff et al., 1984, p. 124). In any case, there was clearly more at issue here than the scientific evidence itself. As Douglas and Wildavsky argue, the level of risk held to be acceptable is a social construct, combining scientific knowledge and values (1983, pp. 4-5). Even if there had been a greater degree of consensus over 'the facts' here - and scientific disagreement is endemic in areas such as these (Douglas and Wildavsky, 1983, chapt. 3) - there would have been disagreement about the acceptability of risks. On the one hand, the government gave more weight to growth, profitability, controlling public expenditure, and the maintenance of good relationships with businesses which it had to regulate, its values being underpinned by a 'business as usual' conception of the economy: on the other hand, critics both in the environmental movement and the medical profession gave more weight to the environment and to health. In the next section I will show how water privatisation created a political space within which the government's critics were able to politicise the debate.

Water privatisation and the debate over water quality

Before their privatisation in 1989, the ten regional water authorities, set up in 1974 alongside the remaining private water companies, had controlled the full water cycle, from extraction through to purification, sewage treatment and disposal (Kinnersley, 1988, chapt. 8). Beside this, they were responsible for policing emissions into the river system. The first Thatcher government inherited from the Labour Party the problem of implementing part two of the *Control of Pollution Act* of 1974 (COPA). The aim of this part of the act was to bolster the powers of the water authorities to clean up inland rivers and to extend their control to estuaries and beaches. The general British principle of attempting to achieve voluntary agreement with polluters (Vogel, 1986) had also been in operation in relation to water quality. Environmentalists argued that the form of control adopted, based on River Quality Objectives rather than absolute limits on pollution, had little scientific justification, objectives being tailored in an ad hoc way to fit the existing levels of pollution (e.g. Cook, 1989, pp. 22-3). Many consents to emit pollution, especially into estuaries, had still not been re-examined in the light of the COPA (Environment Select Committee, 1987, p. xxxvii). Prosecution of those violating consents were very rare and fines were small (Environment Select Committee, 1987, p. xxi).

Influenced by the neo-liberal argument that environmental regulation is a barrier to economic growth and efficiency - a sop to environmentalist special interests (Ward and Samways, 1991) - Thatcher's governments went further than Labour governments in the 1970s towards relaxing the regulatory regime which existed on paper. Despite severe pollution in many rivers and estuaries, notably the Mersey, because of public expenditure constraints, successive Labour governments delayed the implementation of COPA, and the new Conservative government did the same (Pearce, 1986). In part the Conservatives' desire to delay implementation was the result of pressure from large industrial polluters and from the National Farmer's Union (NFU). However, the government also wished to keep down the capital spending of the water authorities in order to minimise public sector borrowing and as part of the Thatcherite programme to make management in nationalised industries operate more like that in the private sector. Under the *Water Act* of 1983 the National Water Council - the government's statutory adviser on water quality issues and an important forum for the coordination of a national water policy - was abolished, partly as a victim of the government's drive against quangos, but also because of pressure from industry. The government turned, instead, to large industrial polluters for advice on water quality (Pearce, 1986, p. 234). At the same time, local authority representation on water authority boards was ended, environmentalists claiming that some authorities were packed with representatives of industry and agriculture. The operation of the boards became much less publicly accessible. This process enabled delayed implementation of COPA to go largely unnoticed.

Because of the government's control of the water authorities' borrowing and pressure to keep water rates down there was a significant squeeze on investment (Environment Select Committee, 1987, pp. xvi-xvii; Kinnersley, 1988, p. 205). The effects of the squeeze were felt both in terms of job losses and in declining standards of pollution control in relation to the water industry's own emissions. Many sewage works exceeded statutory emission limits because of lack of staff, breakdowns, and lack of processing capacity. Emissions of sewage are an important source of pollution because of the phosphates, toxic heavy metals, nitrates and industrial and agricultural chemicals they contain. Not only can this lead to deterioration of environmental quality in rivers but also, because around 70 per cent of drinking water is abstracted from surface waters in Britain, it can feed pollutants back into our drinking water. In order to avoid prosecutions under COPA, the government relaxed discharge consents for 1800 out of the 6600 sewage works between 1980 and 1988, a further 1000 relaxations occurring in the year before privatisation. Even so, many sewage works violated their consents. For instance, figures provided by the Water Authorities Association to the Commons Select Committee on the Environment suggest that in

1986 22 per cent of sewage works failed to meet the requirement to keep within their consents 95 per cent of the time (Environment Select Committee, 1987, p. xvi). Although it was highly critical of the water industry at times, HM's Inspectorate of Pollution, being very dependant upon Water Authority expertise and testing facilities, did not have the resources independently to monitor the increasing number of water authority applications to relax pollution controls. Under COPA, public registers were supposed to be maintained showing the requirements of the discharge consents issued and the results of monitoring. Both Labour and Conservative governments delayed the implementation of this part of the act, one motive for Thatcher's governments being to save political embarrassment over the water authorities' own contribution to pollution (Kinnersley, 1988, p. 122). In the light of this, the lack of separation of regulatory powers due to the conflict of interest between the water authorities' regulatory role and the increased role their plant played in water pollution became an important, and contentious issue (Kinnersley, 1988, chapt. 8; Environment Select Committee, 1987, pp. xix-xx).

Privatisation of the water industry was not seriously discussed in government circles until 1985. Even then, it looked as if only some water authorities would be sold off, Thames Water, which had actually been making a positive return to the Treasury, being a prime candidate. Although fear of future price rises was important, the privatisation debate largely centered upon environmental and related public health issues: the state of rivers, estuaries, and beaches; fears that sales of water authority land would lead to loss of public access and to environmental degradation; and further deterioration of drinking water quality. The government's claim was that privatisation would liberate the industry to invest in pollution control, but the public was not persuaded.

The passage of the *Water Bill* through the House of Commons in late 1988 and 1989 was commonly seen as a public relations disaster for the government as compared to earlier privatisations (Cook, 1989, chapt. 12; Gordon, 1989, chapt. 12). A MORI poll conducted in December 1988 showed that there was a large majority against water privatisation, only 15 per cent being in favour and 75 per cent against (Cook, 1989, p. 90). Given the public opinion data, it is not possible to gauge the degree to which opposition to the privatisation was due to water quality and health issues rather than other bases of concern, although these were clearly significant. What I can do, however, is to follow through in more detail the debates on water quality, both in the run up to privatisation and during the privatisation process itself. I will look at the broad campaigns mounted by pressure groups then focus again upon nitrates, pesticides and lead.

As the 1987/8 report of HM's Inspectorate of Pollution acknowledged, the quality of British rivers had noticeably worsened in the 1980s. As we saw above, the 1985 EC directive on the quality of drinking water lays down guide levels and maximum admissible concentrations for a number of pollutants, including nitrates, pesticide residues, industrial chemicals and solvents, and metals, including lead. The government's failure to meet some EC standards for drinking water and bathing beaches gave much increased leverage to Greenpeace and Friends of the Earth, even though Britain was far from being the only EC member in breach of the directives. A great deal of symbolic play was made by juxtaposing Britain's dirty water and beaches with the image that we had once had the cleanest water in Europe. Not only were environmental groups able to rouse public opinion by drawing attention to the failure to meet standards, but they were also able to apply pressure in Brussels. For instance, a formal complaint over nitrate levels made by Friends of the Earth led the Commission to require a detailed explanation of the government's position in 1987 (Conrad, 1990, p. 31). The British government fought a rearguard action against the EC, at first to keep public expenditure down, then to make the water industry look more attractive to investors. Similarly, the government sought to evade EC directives on the quality of bathing beaches announced in 1976, largely because of the very high capital costs of investing in sewage treatment as compared to pumping effluent out to sea via short outfalls. The effect of pressure group campaigns like this was to alert public opinion to a broad range of environmental and water quality problems, including those over nitrates.

Although increasing levels of nitrates were first noticed in drinking water in the 1970s, particularly in the drought year of 1976, the issue of nitrates was, in effect, off the public political agenda until the run up to privatisation (Hill et al., 1989; Conrad, 1990, pp. 29-33). Although it well knew that the EC directive on nitrate levels in drinking water would come into force in 1985, in line with its general policy the British government at first did little or nothing. Indeed, research into the solution of the problem of nitrate pollution was even cut back in the 1980s. On the basis of the derogations from the EC directive given to water authorities, it has been calculated that in 1985 921,000 consumers drank water which had levels of nitrates exceeding the EC maximum (Conrad, 1990, p. 12), and government figures show that limits had been exceeded at some time during 1987 for 1.6m consumers (FoE, 1990, p. 21).

Although several Member States had already been taken to court over drinking water standards, Nicholas Ridley at first believed that no specific plans to meet EC targets would have to be written into the *Water Bill*, thus preserving the confidence of investors. However, the European Commission took a very tough line, demanding that specific investment plans for the water industry to meet current EC standards on nitrates, pesticides, lead and other pollutants by 1993 should be made available before privatisation. With regard to nitrates, which were commonly seen as the most pressing problem, some short term headway can be made by mixing water from different sources. However, very large investment in de-nitrification plant will eventually be needed to meet EC limits, especially in East Anglia (Conrad, 1990, p. 12). Anglia Water estimates that the consequence may be real cost increases to consumers of between 10 and 27 per cent (Gordon, 1989, p. 149).

Fearing for the successful floatation of the industry because of the costs involved in controlling nitrate and other pollutants, water authorities lobbied hard for longer deadlines. Facing defeat in the House of Lords and the possible delay of the sell off, the government wrote specific targets into the legislation. It activated powers under COPA to control farmers' use of nitrates by designating nitrate sensitive areas near ten water supply sources. Subsequently the DoE seems partially to have accepted the environmentalists case. This was one of the reasons for the increasing tensions between the DoE and MAFF which manifested themselves in the 1980s. Unlike some other agriculture ministries in Europe (Environment Select Committee, 1987, pp. xxix-xxx), MAFF, backed by agribusiness interests, continued to claim that the problems were largely ones of inappropriate agricultural practices, both in relation to fertiliser application and in other areas. Perhaps as a result of this internal conflict, the government intends to rely in the first instance on voluntary compliance with compensation for loss of crops and subsidies for conversion of arable into grazing land. There are worries about the take up rate among farmers and, thus, the effectiveness of the scheme (FoE, 1990, p. 22). No specific penalties for misuse of nitrates were written into the legislation, and the government avoided measures like a nitrate tax which would have had a broad effect on the environment right across Britain and beyond the specific issue of drinking water quality.

There are strong parallels here with the debate on pesticides and lead, the role of the EC again being significant. Between July 1985 and June 1987 Friends of the Earth carried out a survey of water samples which showed that EC maximum acceptable concentrations of 16 pesticides were exceeded for 298 water sources and supplies, with geographical concentrations reflecting the pattern of high use in some arable farming areas (Lees and McVeigh, 1988). Coming in the run up to privatisation, this survey occasioned a great deal of unfavourable press and media comment. The government's response was to attempt to put pressure on the EC to lower what it saw as blanket limits, while granting permissions for some privatised water authorities to carry on supplying water in violation of EC limits up to the year 2000. However, as in the case of nitrates, the British government's case carried little weight in the EC, especially given FoE's application for European judicial review of the government's move to allow the privatised companies to do nothing in the short run. Indeed, EC legislation on pesticides was moving in the opposite direction to that desired by the British government.

The 1985 *Food and Environment Protection Act*, which replaced a voluntary code of practice between MAFF and pesticide producers, was a measure brought largely at the insistence of the EC Commission, which saw the British system as providing a relatively easy regulatory ride, potentially in violation of EC competition policy (FoE, 1990, pp. 78-9). However, there is room to doubt whether this act is a turning point. Proposed EC limits on pesticide residues in potatoes and leaf vegetables were never implemented in Britain. MAFF continues to resist testing of older pesticides, despite some of them being banned in the US. A strong rearguard action has also been fought to try to keep under wraps the operation of various scientific advisory groups on food quality and the safety of agrichemicals. Nevertheless, the politicisation of this area will make it much more difficult for British governments to avoid tougher licensing, stronger regulation of pesticide use, and control of pesticide levels in water.

The story in relation to lead in drinking water is similar to that of nitrates and pesticides. At first the government sought to delay implementation of the 1985 EC directive, many Scottish supplies still being above EC limits in 1989, despite the extension of earlier programs to treat water so as to reduce the problem. In the light of this, environmental groups were able to make a good deal out of the further shift in the position of the government's own advisers who, in line with developments in expert opinion in the US, reported in 1989 that the present EC/UK standard was, in any case, too lax (FoE, 1990, p. 25).

The debates on nitrates, pesticides and lead fed into the debate on the environmental regulation of the water industry after privatisation. The DoE's 1986 privatisation white paper had envisaged selling off the water authorities as they stood, so that the privatised companies would continue to combine their existing regulatory role with that of water utilities. Although some individuals within the water industry were critical of this approach, the water authorities collectively supported this option (Kinnersley, 1988, p. 132), further reinforcing the dislike of Thatcher's government for new regulatory quangos. However, the delay of the privatisation process caused by the 1987 election allowed opponents of this move to exert pressure upon Nicholas Ridley for a different regulatory structure. In the event the new National Rivers Authority (NRA) became responsible for the quality of rivers, while HM's Inspectorate of Pollution monitors drinking water quality. It might seem, then, that the new regime was simply a victory for the environmental groups concerned about water quality, particularly the Council for the Protection of Rural England (CPRE). However, although the CPRE was one factor, both the EC Commission and large industrial polluters were very loth to accept the government's original idea. The most significant factor was probably that the initial proposal violated EC competition law.

Potentially the NRA has the institutional autonomy and independent expertise to act more toughly. Moreover, when it comes to regulating the water industry itself, the pricing and competition watch-dog for the privatised water industry may link price levels of individual companies to the meeting of quality standards, thus providing additional regulatory teeth. There are also indications that the NRA is trying to establish a tougher reputation. By the end of 1990 the NRA had either brought prosecutions, or had prosecutions pending, against all ten privatised water companies (Environment Digest, Oct 1990). The number of prosecutions of farmers polluting rivers has been stepped up, especially in the west of England, and some exemplary prosecutions of large industrial polluters have been pushed through - the prosecution of Shell UK over a major oilspill in the Mersey being the most visible. Furthermore, the NRA has proposed automatic monitoring in order more rigidly to enforce existing standards written into the 140,000 permissions to pollute it inherited from the water authorities' regulatory regime. However, despite these clear signals, there are doubts about the NRA's ability to deliver better results.

Just like other environmental regulatory agencies, under Thatcher governments the NRA was chronically short of money and manpower, and this greatly reduced the chances that policies would actually be implemented. In the summer of 1990 the NRA made urgent requests to the DoE for greater resources. It claimed that unless the shortfall in resources (which it estimated might be over £100m by 1994) was made good, there was no chance of cleaning up Britain's rivers. One token of the problem is that the NRA cannot afford to monitor emissions from sewage works at weekends, a fact that several water companies are known to take advantage of. At local level the NRA is still very dependent on the water companies for laboratory facilities. Moreover, there has been some talk in John Major's government about disbanding the NRA and merging its functions with those of HM's Pollution Inspectorate. Although this may make some sense in terms of integrating regulation, the suspicion is that some major polluters do not like the NRA's tougher line and would welcome its demise.

The 'Green Dowry' of £6 billion promised to the water industry right at the end of the passage of the *Water Bill* through Parliament was designed to facilitate the industry's sell off in the face of very adverse reaction by the City to the likely future costs of clean-up. It has been estimated that in order to meet existing EC drinking water standards a capital investment of £2 billion is needed over the next four years while capital investment of £20 billion may be needed over the next twenty years to replace ageing treatment plant and sewers. Following on from the rapid price increases in the lead up to privatisation, the price increases of 5 per cent over the rate of inflation allowed by the government for the 1990s, which are designed to cover these investment costs, mean that the real price of water will increase very rapidly. In 1990 the DoE lost the cabinet battle for pollution taxes against a coalition of the Treasury, MAFF, the Department of Transport and the Department of Trade and Industry (Ward and Samways, 1991). The idea was not emphasised in the government's 1990 white paper *This Common Inheritance*, which is supposed to set the environmental agenda for the decade. Like the Green Dowry, the planned price increases protect the profitability of the water industry and polluters while imposing costs on consumers, the poorest suffering the most in relative terms.

Conclusion

As I showed above, there is considerable expert disagreement over the health threat posed by drinking water quality. It is difficult, if not impossible, to come up with reliable predictions of the expected number of deaths caused by long-term exposure to small doses of pollutants in drinking water. In contrast, we have relatively hard figures for the number of people who die each year through smoking-related diseases or in car accidents. Despite the uncertainties, many would conclude that drinking water is one of the lesser threats. For example, in relation to cancer, Doll and Peto argue that, while the largest risks probably stem from dietary factors:

> it is probable that the most important [dietary factors] would turn out not to be ingestion of powerful carcinogens or pre-carcinogens...but rather nutritional factors, ranging from gross aspects of diet to vitamins, trace elements and other micro-nutrients which may either enhance or inhibit carcinogenesis (1981, p. 1258).

While the authors explicitly warn against ingestion of carcinogens and their precursors from dietary sources (1981, p. 1258), their judgement seems to be that these are unimportant as compared to, say, smoking (1981, p. 1257, table 21).

The sorts of provisional conclusions reached by Doll and Peto might seem to suggest that those participants in the US debate on water quality who see massive investments in clean-up as an irrational use of health resources are correct. Some in the US also accuse the environmental movement of manipulating fear of cancer in order to get water clean-up for broader environmental reasons. (1) The related conclusion here might be that, drawing on British cultural biases about clean water together with fears over such diseases as cancer, environmentalists used a unique political opportunity structure provided by the interaction of the EC and the privatisation process to foist investments which are irrational in health terms on the British public.

There are a number of reasons why such a conclusion, based on an analysis of acceptable risk, might be over-simplistic. (2) It could be argued that the decisions here are not made under risk (where accurate 'objective' probabilities can be defined) or even under uncertainty (where there is enough information for individuals to make subjective risk estimates). In relation to nitrates, pesticides and lead we are radically short of information, as I showed above. In such contexts some have suggested that it is rational to use a conservative, minimax criterion which assumes the worst consequence for each potential course of action and picks that course with the 'best worst-case' payoff. Given the long latency periods, the 'worst case' might be an epidemic of water-related cancers in future years, something which cannot be contemplated. Another argument is that individuals' utility functions are not linear in risk levels as assessed by experts. Rather they exhibit risk aversion. Either form of negative reaction to risk would be viewed as rational by some economists. (3) Secondly, it is not unreasonable for people's attitudes to differ between risks they 'choose' to take, such as smoking or eating cream cakes, and risks they cannot really avoid, such as drinking what comes out of the tap (Starr, 1969; but c.f Douglas and Wildavsky, 1982, pp. 16-21). Thirdly, as I showed above, water quality in Britain was becoming measurably worse in the 1980s. Even if health risks are currently low, it may sometimes be rational to invest to prevent them becoming worse (Fischhoff et al., 1984, p. 127), although this will depend partly on how much weight is placed on the future, as well as anticipated future risks.

My feeling is that such justifications are not enough. If they apply to drinking water quality they obviously apply with at least as much force to numerically larger dietary and environmental sources of the same carcinogens and heavy metals which we ingest in drinking water. In preventive health terms it would probably be more rational to spend money on eliminating other sources first. Moreover, the same sorts of argument would seem to apply to, say, the looming AIDS epidemic among heterosexuals: strictly in health terms, similar arguments suggest we might better spend our money preventing this. However, as I have emphasised all along, we cannot separate health issues from broader environmental issues here. Investment could be justified when environmental benefits are added in.

One problem here is that mixing water to get rid of nitrates, investing in de-nitrification plant, using filters to get rid of pesticide residues, and so on hardly seems the rational solution environmentally. Such measures, besides being expensive, do nothing to save the countryside from the depredations of modern agriculture. Surely the rational long-term course of action in the light of massive EC food surpluses and environmental decline in the countryside would either be to tax use of nitrates and pesticides down to low levels or to legislate against their over-use. (Of course, the pollution of groundwaters might necessitate the use of some technical fixes in the short-term). Similar 'polluter pays' measures might be applied to industry. As I showed above, this course is currently blocked by the combination of business interests and political distrust.

A second problem is that economic considerations might override environmental ones. The claim of agribusiness in relation to pesticides and fertilisers is that a 'polluter pays' approach would massively increase food prices, destroying the industry for insignificant environmental gains. But as Sagoff has cogently argued (1988), we may proceed as a society even if a social cost-benefit analysis which includes the monetary values individuals place upon the benefits they, themselves, derive from environmental clean-up leads to the conclusion that this is unjustified. The process of political deliberation and debate can lead to a public consensus that something should be done. This becomes embodied in our broader 'ethical' preferences, which show non-individualistic concern for the current well-being of society as a whole and for its future, as well as concern for nature as an end-in-itself, not a source of human benefits. It may be that there is a such consensus in Britain over water quality. (4)

Arguments like those of Sagoff undercut the individualistic and anthropocentric ethics of much environmental cost-benefit analysis. But, as Sagoff himself concedes (1988, chapt. 9), opportunity costs must still get factored into the political process. In a well known article Anthony Downs pictures an issue attention cycle in environmental politics (1978): gloomy prognoses by informed insiders, often in environmental groups, leads to an expert debate, a rise in media and public attention, public mobilisation, and policy change: but as the policy changes begin to be implemented, the costs become apparent to the public, leading to a counter reaction and partial failure to implement the legislation. Clearly the 'up' phase of Downs' model is a reasonable schematic representation of water politics in the 1980s. We should be concerned that the present public consensus will be dissolved by an individualistic counter-reaction, based on the unfair way in which costs are being socially distributed and the inefficient technical fixes chosen for problems which are better treated at their root.

Footnotes

1) The US debate is covered by Douglas and Wildavsky (1982, pp. 50-60). As pointed out by these authors, the work of Doll and Peto was seen as quite contentious by many in the US.

2) Schwarz and Thompson provide a useful summary critique of risk assessment written from a 'social construction of science and technology' perspective (1990, chapt. 7).

3) The minimax criterion (and the related minimax regret criterion) are far from being universally accepted by economists and philosophers. The basic objection is that there is no rational justification for always assuming the worst, except in situations which resemble zero-sum games.

4) An unfortunate aspect of Sagoff's book is that he seems to picture the US political and legal systems as relatively bias-free and open, and the American political tradition as unproblematic. His argument would have more weight if political life in the US more closely approached a Habermasian ideal speech community (Dryzek, 1986, chapt. 15). While making no claim that the water debate in Britain approached this ideal, I think it was open enough for Sagoff's approach to be brought to bear.

Bibliography/references

Agriculture Select Committee (1987), *HC 379-1. The Effects of Pesticides on Human Health Vol. 1*, HMSO, London.
Conrad, J. (1990), *Nitrate Pollution and Politics*, Gower, Aldershot.

Cook, J. (1989), *Dirty Water*, Unwin, London.

DHSS (Department of Health and Social Security) (1980), *Lead and Health*, HMSO, London.

DoE (Department of the Environment) (1977), *Lead In Drinking Water*, HMSO, London.

Doll, R. and Peto, R. (1981), *The Causes of Cancer*, Oxford University Press, Oxford.

Douglas, M. and Wildavsky, A. (1982), *Risk and Culture*, University of California Press, Berkeley.

Downs, A. (1972), 'Up and Down With Ecology: the Issue Attention Cycle', *Public Interest*, vol. 28, pp. 38-50.

Dryzek, J. (1986), *Rational Ecology*, Blackwell, Oxford.

Dudley, N. (1990), *Nitrates: The Threat to Food and Water*, Merlin, London.

Ellis, K. (1989), *Surface Water Pollution and Its Control*, Macmillan, London.

Environment Select Committee (1987), *HC183-I Pollution of Rivers and Estuaries vol.1*, HMSO, London.

Fischhoff, B., Watson, S. and Hope, C. (1984), 'Defining Risk', *Policy Sciences*, vol. 17, 123-39.

Friends of the Earth (1990), *How Green is Britain: The Government's Environmental Record*, Hutchinson, London.

Gordon, S. (1989), *Down the Drain*, Macdonald, London.

Hill, M., Aaronovitch, S. and Baldock, D. (1989), 'Non-Decision Making in Pollution Control In Britain: Nitrate Pollution, the EEC Drinking Water Directive and Agriculture', *Policy and Politics*, vol. 17, 227-40.

Illich, I. (1985), H_2O *and the Waters of Forgetfullness*, Marian Boyars, London.

Kinnersley, D. (1988), *Troubled Waters*, Hilary Shipman, London.

Landsdown, R. and Yule, W. (eds.) (1986), *The Lead Debate*, Croom Helm, London.

Lees, A. and McVeigh, K. (1988), *An Investigation of Pesticide Pollution In Drinking Water in England and Wales*, FoE, London.

McCormick, J. (1991), *British Politics and the Environment*, Earthscan, London.

Moore, M. (1986), 'Sources of Lead Exposure', in, Landsdown, R. and Yule, W. (eds), *The Lead Debate*, Croom Helm, London.

OECD (1986), *Water Pollution By Fertilizers and Pesticides*, OECD, Paris.

Pearce, F. (1986), `Dirty Water Under the Bridge', in, Goldsmith, E. and Hilyard, N. (eds), *Green Britain or Industrial Wasteland*, Polity, Cambridge.

Price, B. (1986), 'Lead Astray', in, Goldsmith, E. and Hilyard, N. (eds), *Green Britain or Industrial Wasteland*, Polity, Cambridge.

Rosenbaum, W. (1991), *Environmental Politics and Policy (2nd. ed.)*, Congressional Quarterly Press, Washington.

Royal Commission on Environmental Pollution (1983), *Ninth Report: Lead in the Environment*, HMSO, London.

Sagoff, M. (1988), *The Economy of the Earth*, Cambridge University Press, Cambridge.

Schwarz, M. and Thompson, M. (1990), *Divided We Stand*, Harvester/Wheatsheaf, Hemel-Hempstead.

Starr, C. (1969), 'Social Benefit Versus Technological Risk: What Is Our Society Willing To Pay For Safety', *Science*, vol. 165, 1232-8.

Vogel, D. (1986), *National Styles of Regulation: Environmental Policing in Great Britain and the United States*, Cornell University Press, Ithaca.

Ward, H. and Samways, D. (1991), 'Environmental Policy', in, Marsh, D. and Rhodes, R. (eds.), *Implementing Thatcherite Policies: Audit of an Era*, Open University Press, Buckingham.

Ward, H. with Samways, D., and Benton, T. (1990), 'Environmental Politics and Policy', in, Dunleavy, P. , Gamble, A. and Peele, G. (eds), *Developments in British Politics 3*, Macmillan, London.

Wilson, D. (1983), *The Lead Scandal*, Heinemann, London.

9 Prevention from above? The role of the European Community

Elizabeth Bomberg and John Peterson

Since the mid-1980s, the influence of the European Community (EC) has increased in a range of policy debates related to health and the quality of life. The EC was created as an essentially economic community with no firm legal basis for dealing with such issues. More recently, especially since the acceptance of the Single European Act (SEA) in 1987, the EC's role has expanded to the point where it now prods its Member States towards preventive strategies in a host of policy sectors.

It is difficult to generalise about EC preventive policies. 'Prevention' is not a discrete policy sector. Rather, it is a *strategy* which is evident in a range of EC policies. Studying the way in which the EC promotes and embraces preventive strategies involves examining 'corners' of numerous and varied policy sectors. The policies which are the focus for this chapter may appear to be peripheral to both the EC's core economic policies or its Member States' core national health policies. There is no 'EC health policy' *per se*.

However, if prevention is viewed as a strategy, then the EC may be seen as having developed a distinct set of preventive policies. These policies can be defined as those which seek to eliminate or manage risks which could otherwise have adverse effects on human health or the environment. Preventive strategies are most evident in EC policies for the environment, consumers, social rights and research and development (R&D).

As the EC's competencies in these policy areas have expanded, so have the conflicts surrounding 'preventive issues'. The key determinants of EC preventive policies are often rivalries between Community institutions or disputes between them and the individual Member States over the EC's proper policy role. Most EC policies cross over several departments of the European Commission, the EC's 'civil service.'

Even when the Commission pursues a unified strategy toward a common end, resistance or non-compliance is frequent at the national level where policies are implemented. Conflict is thus often multi-dimensional.

Despite this complexity, the EC embraces long-term preventive strategies far more often than do its constituent Member States. Two factors are crucial in explaining why. First, the EC's central institutions - particularly the Commission but also the European Parliament (EP) - have had considerable success in pushing preventive strategies onto the EC's agenda. Both have insisted that the EC needs truly common preventive policies in the name of both the internal market and the general improvement of the quality of life in western Europe. Preventive strategies serve the self-interests of the Commission and EP because expanded EC policies in these sectors means more power for EC institutions in European policy making. Second, the undemocratic, technocratic nature of the EC as a policy making system is well suited to long-term, preventive strategies. Key EC actors (such as the Commission) are not constrained by short-term electoral considerations as are national governments.

This chapter begins by tracing the development of a legal basis for EC preventive policies. Section II examines the policy making machinery of the EC, emphasising its fragmented character. The complex dynamics of the wider political setting within which EC preventive policies are made is the focus for section III. Four case studies of EC policies for water quality, auto emissions, food hygiene and tobacco advertising are presented in section IV. The conclusion compares the EC as a system for policy making with British government and seeks to explain why the EC increasingly embraces preventive strategies where its Member States cannot or will not.

I. The development of EC competence

The original Treaty of Rome contained no provisions for common environmental or health policies. Yet, as the Single European Act (SEA) was debated between 1985-7, concerns arose that the increased trade and economic activity generated by the internal market could have undesirable effects on the environment and public health. Fears also emerged that workers' rights might be threatened after the free movement of capital was secured. Governments would have new incentives to reduce social benefits as they competed to attract businesses which might seek to locate and invest where labour costs were cheapest.

Thus, the SEA included numerous provisions for ensuring that preventive policies could be enacted as the internal market was constructed. The Rome Treaty was amended so that nearly all legislation related to the internal market would be authorised by qualified majority voting. This change made it impossible for one Member State to veto legislation. Implicitly, the new article also was meant to serve as the basis for environmental legislation since many 'environmental protection measures also have objectives and consequences which are directly linked to the functioning of the internal market' (Johnson and Corcelle, 1989, p. 344). For example, firms in Member States which impose minimal penalties on polluters can receive unfair trade advantages. The distortion is eliminated when common EC penalties are adopted.

The SEA also contained an entirely new title which aimed 'to preserve, protect and improve the quality of the environment; and to contribute towards protecting human health'. The title emphasised that to achieve these goals 'preventive action should be taken ... environmental damage should be rectified at the source'. It also required that any Commission proposal which in any way concerned health, safety, the environment or consumers should take as a base a high level of protection (CEC, 1990d, p. 5). Moreover, Member States were given the right to institute national environmental or worker health and safety regulations which were stricter than EC laws (Corbett, 1987, p. 250).

Yet, the acceptance of legislation proposed under the new title still required unanimity on the EC's Council of Ministers. The upshot was that the EC received a new legal mandate to put into action environmental and certain social policies. But unless proposals could be clearly linked to the proper functioning of the internal market, all Member States had to agree on both their methods and goals.

Other articles of the SEA made possible EC legislation on working environments and worker health and safety. These measures required only qualified majorities on the Council to be made law. However, all other health and social policies had to be made unanimously.

In short, the SEA represented a clear shift of legislative power to the EC in areas ripe for new preventive strategies. It redefined the Community as an institution with policy concerns beyond economic growth and prosperity. By providing a sounder constitutional footing, it ushered in a period of increased EC activism in preventive policy making.

The Treaty on Political Union agreed at Maastricht in December 1991 further strengthened the EC's mandate to legislate in areas of preventive policy. If ratified, the Maastricht treaty would sanction majority voting rather than unanimity on the 'cross-border aspects' of environmental policy (i.e. the transport of toxic wastes). More generally, the treaty would change legislative procedures for many preventive policies. The Commission would be given wider scope to propose new policies related to health, consumer protection, research and development (R&D) and environmental strategy. The EP would be granted increased powers of veto or co-decision with the Council on these same issues.

Elsewhere, the results of Maastricht were disappointing to advocates of expanded EC preventive policies. A proposal to subject to majority voting rules on working conditions and information on employee health risks was blocked by the UK. The negotiations led to a bizarre 'social protocol' which allowed the UK to 'opt in' to new EC policies, but remain unbound by any which it opposed. Proposals to include in the Treaty a reference to the EC's 'federal vocation' were voted down. Instead, the Treaty highlighted the principle of subsidiarity, which mandates Community action 'only if and in so far as the objectives of the proposed action cannot be sufficiently achieved by Member States and can therefore by reason of the scale or effects of the proposed action, be better achieved by the Community' (Council of the European Communities and CEC, 1992, pp. 13-4). Earlier, the SEA invoked the same principle in its Title on the environment: 'The Community shall take action relating to the environment to the extent to which the objectives [of EC policy] can be attained better at the Community level than at the level of the individual Member States' (Butterworths European Information Services, 1989, p. 173).

The subsidiarity principle is double-edged. On one hand, it provides a powerful justification for the EC to develop policies where it has never done so before. On the other, it places limits on EC action. The EC should only be involved in areas of policy where it can provide some sort of advantage or 'added value' to existing national policies. All Member States can agree on the logic of a principle which is so vague, but it leaves wide open the question of precisely where EC policies bring advantages over purely national ones. The broad implication is that the extent of the EC's competence in a range of preventive policy areas will continue to be a major bone of contention in the 1990s.

II. The EC's machinery for preventive policy

Diffuse issues

Environmental policy is where the EC's 'preventive powers' are most pronounced. The EC passed more environmental legislation between 1989 and 1991 than in the previous 20 years combined. Key issues on the EC's legislative agenda include controlling risks related to chemicals, protecting natural resources and combating water, air and noise pollution.

Recently, the Community's strategy has shifted towards the greater use of economic and fiscal incentives to protect the environment (see EP, 1990). In 1991, the Commission proposed a tax on all non-renewable sources of energy, together with a levy on fuels emitting carbon dioxide (CO_2). Although rejected by the Council, the proposal was indicative of new thinking within the Commission on environmental protection. The EC's 'Eco-Label,' which was due to appear in late 1992, was another attempt to develop a market solution to the problem of promoting environmentally friendly behaviour. The label was designed to counter exaggerated, misleading or unfounded claims that products are environmentally-friendly.

Consumer policy covers food quality and product safety. The EC is concerned with control of food additives and the healthy preparation and packaging of goods. Specifically, the EC has passed directives governing the labelling of food, hygienic processing and packaging (i.e. in slaughterhouses), and regulations monitoring the effects of certain foods on health (i.e. the health effects of fruit grown using pesticides).

EC consumer legislation is incomplete. Consumer organisations such as the Consumers in the EC Group (CECG) complain there are not yet enough common EC-wide rules to make sure goods are safe. For instance, children's toys are covered by one directive but many other child hazards (nursery furniture, sporting goods) are not (Crampton and Eversley, 1990, p. 80).

Social policy has come to be seen as a necessary element of the internal market programme by the Commission, the EP and Member States such as Germany and Denmark. Interest in extending the EC's competence was reflected in the acceptance (by all Member States except the UK) at the Madrid summit of 1989 of the Social Charter. The Charter was a 'non-binding and heavily diluted declaration of principles (which) papered over a great deal of dissension' (Rhodes, 1991, p. 246), but it did commit Member States to develop common EC rules on working hours, fair and reasonable wages, the protection of children and adolescents, etc.

Political enthusiasm for the Social Charter waned considerably and quickly after its passage. The high costs and dubious feasibility of achieving goals such as 'equitable wages', combined with the need for unanimity, led to agreement on little besides legislation related to workplace health and safety. In 1991, a cross-party UK Commons Employment Committee report concluded that the Social Charter was merely a 'propaganda pipe dream' (quoted in *The Independent*, 21 August 1991). It remains to be seen whether and how the Maastricht Treaty's new social protocol will work. However, the Commission and EP are determined to push new social policies onto the EC's agenda and now have a stronger legal basis to do so.

EC spending on *collaborative R&D* into biotechnology, a science with major impacts for health care and medicine, was increased by one-third in the 1990-94 budget (Peterson, 1989). Specific programmes seek to develop environmentally-friendly inputs for agriculture and improve food safety (CEC, 1990a; CEC, 1990c, p. 79-84). Funding for environmental R&D was doubled in 1989 and the EC began to group together these funds with those for research into genetic engineering, radiation protection, and medicine/health. The intent was to create a single tranche of funding for improving the quality of life in Europe. The Commission's interest in new preventive strategies is aptly illustrated by its programme for 'socio-economic environmental research' (SEER). SEER funds research on the 'societal causes of environmental degradation (and) measures for prevention' (CEC, 1990f, p. 1). The Commission's proposal for SEER explains:

> The last few years have created a common understanding that dealing with environmental problems requires preventive rather than end-of-pipe abatement strategies. Likewise it is being understood that - although the development of clean or green technologies is a most important agenda - technology cannot be expected to bring about all solutions necessary: a number of fundamental causes of pollution and environmental degradation lies [sic] within the organisation and function of society itself (CEC, 1990f, p. 1).

The proposal reflects a new awareness within the Commission of the links between the EC's various policies for the environment, agriculture, consumers, R&D, etc. Integrating strategies across policy sectors is critical for a 'preventive ethos' to make its presence felt at the EC level generally. However, as the next section will show, the difficulties of pursuing such broad strategies at the EC level are formidable.

Diffuse institutions: fragmentation and competition

While the SEA mandated that environmental and consumer concerns needed to be considered in all other areas of EC policy (Freestone, 1991, p. 137), the EC's institutional structure mitigates against such an integrated approach. The EC's 17 Commissioners are national political appointees who must in theory renounce any loyalties to their own country and serve only the 'general European interest'. Yet, this does not make them a collegial body in the same sense as the British cabinet is collegial. Commissioners bring national orientations and political links to their posts which are never entirely abandoned.

Different sections of the Commission are often set in conflict with one another in much the same way as are ministries in national settings. Most preventive issues cross over the policy responsibilities of multiple Directorates-General (DGs), the Brussels equivalent of ministries. The DGs tend to be tightly compartmentalised and often pursue their own bureaucratic missions in isolation from whatever the rest of the Commission is doing. For example, DG III, which is responsible for the single market, is keen to ensure that the setting of high environmental standards by self-proclaimed 'greener' countries does not create new non-tariff barriers to trade. By contrast, the EC's department for environmental and consumer protection (DG XI) is more concerned that the search for common solutions does not yield 'least common denominator' results or 'a half-hearted and ultimately inadequate environmental policy' (CEC, 1990d, p. 6).

Conflict exists not only within the Commission, but also between EC institutions. Although still a consultative rather than legislative body, the EP's role in the legislative process was enhanced by the SEA. Previously, the Council of Ministers needed only to seek the EP's advice on Commission proposals; advice which subsequently could be ignored. Now, much EC legislation - including nearly all related to the internal market - goes to the EP for a 'second reading'. At this stage, with the Commission's approval, the EP can insist on amendments, which can be thrown out by the Council only on a unanimous vote. The Maastricht Treaty, if ratified, would create a new 'codecision' process which would give the EP the right to negotiate amendments directly with the Council and to veto certain types of legislation.

In political terms, the EP has seized upon increasing environmental awareness amongst its electorate. The success of many national Green parties in the 1989 European election helped the EP consolidate its reputation as the most 'green' of all Community institutions. The Parliament's committees regularly conduct their own inquiries into issues such as the handling of waste, water quality, and nuclear safety. The increased constitutional and political power of the EP means that both the Commission and Council must take EP views more seriously.

In short, all EC preventive policies are subject to bargaining between a vast array of actors. This process usually features competition between individual DGs and Commissioners, various EP committees, and representatives of affected interest groups. By nature, each EC institution seeks to preserve or expand its own powers, 'perhaps even if it means reducing the capacity of the resulting arrangements to make "good" community policy' (Peters, 1992, p. 118).

Diffuse patterns of implementation

The implementation of preventive policies accentuates the diffuse nature of the EC's policy process. The EC's most successful policy tool generally has been the directive. Directives are binding only as to the result to be achieved, leaving national authorities to choose forms and methods of application. Thus, EC environmental law can be applied flexibly by developing proposals which accommodate existing national legislation and administrative practices.

The price of such flexibility is often policy incoherence, lax implementation and even outright non-compliance (Liberatore, 1991, p. 290). It is widely agreed that EC environmental law is 'environmentally stringent, comprehensive and far-ranging, but ... also widely flouted' (Anderson, 1991, p. 182).   Close to 400 cases of non-compliance were being pursued by the Commission as of mid-1991.

The Commission's position in enforcing EC legislation is weak.   It lacks any 'green' force of environmental inspectors, and more generally is quite a small bureaucracy which is chronically understaffed in parts of many DGs.   It learns of violations of EC environmental law - or laws related to other preventive policies - only if it receives a complaint from an individual, pressure group or other interested party (often a rival industrial firm).   These 'agents' are more vigilant in some countries than in others.   While the Commission received more complaints about the UK than any other member State in 1990, the UK actually ranked fourth among the EC 12 in having the lowest number of outstanding cases pending for violation of EC environmental rules (see Table 1).

Table 9.1. Outstanding cases of EC environmental law violation - May 1991.

	Warning letters	Reasoned opinions	Court cases	Total
Spain	30	25	11	66
Italy	16	28	9	53
Greece	13	31	6	50
Belgium	3	17	10	30
Germany	1	18	11	30
France	9	13	6	28
Ireland	12	13	3	28
Portugal	8	15	1	24
UK	12	9	2	23
Netherlands	5	15	2	22
Luxembourg	1	11	2	14
Denmark	2	2	0	4

(Source: Unpublished European Commission data cited in *The Economist*, 1991b, p. 54).

European governments at all levels need the expertise and vigilance of watchdog groups and individuals if they hope to enforce preventive policies. The reliance of the EC on nongovernmental organisations to help it monitor compliance with EC 'preventive legislation' is almost total.   This reliance, combined with the heavy caseload of the European Court of Justice (ECJ), explains why an average of about four years (50 months) separates the arrival of a complaint about an alleged violation of an environmental directive and a ruling by the ECJ.

Thus, the EC's machinery for implementing preventive policies - which themselves cut across traditional policy boundaries - is fragmented and complex.   The Commission has almost no independent capacity to implement policies or monitor compliance with them. Moreover, as section III argues, preventive policies often are caught in wider, 'macro-debates' about the EC's general institutional development.

III. Machinations - the wider political setting

The EC is marked by substantial political conflict about the proper line to be drawn between national and EC powers. It was intended that such debates largely would be settled at Maastricht and isolated from the more immediate task of getting on with the 1992 project. Yet, the emphasis of the Maastricht treaty on the subsidiarity principle - a vague idea which begs more questions than it answers - reflects the fact that the negotiations on Political Union 'never had a specific purpose supported by all Member States beyond that of an ill defined "union"' (Bradshaw, 1991, p. 82). The difficulties surrounding ratification of the Maastricht Treaty illustrate this point. Controversy over the extent of the Community's own competence will continue to permeate the day-to-day business of formulating proposed EC preventive policies.

This section first sets out general patterns for agenda-setting and interest mediation in the areas of environmental and social policy. Second, it illustrates how disputes between Member States and broad 'macro-controversies' about the future development of the EC cannot help but mitigate against truly common preventive policies.

Agenda-setting and coalition formation

EC policies for the environment, consumers, social protection and R&D are all quite new. Patterns of agenda-setting and coalition formation still are being established and resist clear or simple characterisations. The fragmentation of EC policy making into different sectors, each with its own distinctive range of actors, imperatives, and Treaty bases, makes the notion of *policy networks* an apt tool for analysing EC decision-making (Peterson, 1991; Boons, 1991; Marsh and Rhodes, 1992). Because of the 'newness' of most EC preventive policies, networks are rarely tightly integrated with established, dominant interests. Thus, the agenda for EC preventive policy making is relatively open and accessible.

Discrete policy networks which correspond to different issue-areas show different actors setting the tone and parameters of EC policy debates. For example, the agenda-setting *nous* of Greens in the EP was demonstrated repeatedly during the late 1980s on a wide range of environmental policy issues (see Bomberg, 1992). The Netherlands has taken a lead role in pushing the Commission to adopt at the EC level the same ambitious and overtly preventive approach reflected in recent Dutch national environmental programmes (Boons, 1991, p. 15). As net contributors to the EC's budget, Germany and the UK have been decisive in determining priorities for EC R&D spending. Each have 'world-class' environmental technology industries and have pushed to increase funds for environmental R&D.

Inevitably, however, analysis of EC agenda-setting and coalition-building in any policy area must begin by considering the role of the Commission. It is not a traditional bureaucracy which simply serves as a tool of elected political masters. Rather, the Commission's political role is sanctioned by the Rome Treaty, which grants it the exclusive right to propose EC legislation. In purely legal terms, this gives the Commission significant agenda-setting powers which national civil services do not enjoy. Yet, a point central to understanding the EC's policy making process is the

Commission's meagre administrative capabilities. One outcome of Maastricht could be that 'the Commission will ... be offered a significant expansion in its responsibilities at a time when it is not clear that it can cope effectively with its current duties' (Bradshaw, 1991, p. 85).

Resource or 'structural' dependencies of this kind are critical variables within policy networks because 'they set the "chessboard" where ... interests manoeuvre for advantage' (Peterson, 1991, p. 272). The dependence of the Commission on outside groups, firms and individuals extends to strategic planning and policy formulation related to a range of preventive policies. For example, writing in the trade journal of the British Town and Country Planning Association (TCPA), the head of DG XI urges: 'The Commission has only a small staff involved in environmental policymaking and depends to a large extent on inputs from bodies such as the TCPA as it develops its policies. We would therefore welcome contributions to the development of our thinking' (Brinkhorst, 1991, p. 21).

Boons (1991, p. 6) argues that the specialist information and expertise provided by CEFIC (*Conseil Europeen des Federations de l'Industries Chimique*) the peak organisation of the European chemical industry, means it 'is often involved in the formulation of EC-policy relevant to the chemical industry'. The CEFIC was intimately involved in the development of a directive passed in 1991 by agricultural ministers which regulated the sale of new types of pesticides. The directive clearly conflicted with an earlier directive approved in 1990 by the Environmental Council of Ministers, which stipulated that genetically-modified organisms (GMOs) designed for use as pesticides could only be sold after a detailed assessment of their environmental impact. The later directive contained no such provisions for assessing GMOs and mandated that a committee of agricultural experts - not environmental authorities - would license new pesticides. Both DG XI and Green MEPs argued that leaving such decisions to a committee associated with agribusiness amounted to the inmates taking over the asylum (see MacKenzie, 1991a). This incident showed how industry groups can exploit the fragmentation of EC power into discrete policy networks, such as those for environmental and agricultural policies.

More generally, the Commission derives much of its authority from its close working links to a broad range of affected interests. Only the Commission can propose preventive policies, but its fragmented structure and lack of resources means that it usually holds no monopoly over the agenda. It must build broad coalitions if EC policies are to be based on a new preventive ethos.

Why 'macro-controversies' permeate preventive policies

The Commission and EP have embraced preventive policies with enthusiasm as means for increasing their own powers. For example, both have fallen upon environmental policy and 'green issues' with some relief. Pollution does not respect national boundaries and its control is clearly a trans-national problem requiring common solutions.

In social policy, the EP often has taken the lead in arguing that the benefits of the internal market must be spread to labour. For example, in 1990 the Socialist group in the EP threatened to block or delay all internal market legislation because it viewed the original draft version of the Social Charter as a sop to the arguments of the UK and industrialists that there was no need for it. On EC R&D spending, the EP and Commission have emphasised the EC's collective competitive weakness in high-tech industries *vis-a-vis* the USA and Japan. Both have 'argu(ed) confidently that if ever there were a case for European integration, this is it' (Duff 1986, p. 48).

Thus, the EP and especially the Commission 'play politics' in preventive policy making and constantly argue that effective policies require increased EC powers and resources. For example, the EC's former Environment Commissioner, Carlo Ripa Di Meana urged that the European Environmental Agency (EEA), created in 1990, develop an EC environmental 'inspectorate' to monitor implementation and compliance by Member States. To concentrate the minds of Member States on the need for such an inspectorate, the Commission issued several ambitious proposals on sewage discharge, animal habitats and pesticide control during 1990-1 which clearly threatened to overload the capacity of the Commission to police EC standards.

Since the passage of the SEA, the Commission has boldly challenged national sovereignty over policies for the environment, consumers, health and safety and R&D at one time or another. The Member State which most often has resisted the Commission's incursions into new realms of preventive policy has been the UK. The 'British problem' has had as much to do with style as the substance of new proposals. For example, in worker and product safety, the notion of enforcing stringent and mandatory pan-European standards of the sort proposed by the Commission is alien to the British civil service, which is used to regulation based on voluntary agreements and 'gentleman's understandings' between government and industry.

However, Spain is by far the Member State which has breached EC environmental rules most often. Spain has no Ministry of the Environment and environmental policy comes under the remit of its Ministry of Public Works. The implementation of EC law is the responsibility of the highly autonomous Spanish regional governments (see *The Economist*, 1991a, 1991b). Generally, the Spanish position is that the stringency of EC regulations hinders economic growth and development. Greece, Portugal and Italy are also inveterate violators of EC environmental laws and tend to take a similar line, although less vocally. A basic cleavage in EC environmental politics is between northern countries who stress legislative, standards-setting measures and the southern countries who favour more expensive spending programmes to remedy problems such as soil erosion, forest fires and coastal pollution (CEC 1990d, p. 17). At Maastricht, the price of substituting majority voting for unanimity in new areas of environmental policy was a new 'cohesion fund', part of which will assist southern Member States in meeting the costs of implementing EC environmental standards (see MacKenzie, 1991b). Still, the north-south divide in the EC has become as perceptible in environmental policy as in any other.

Wider political disputes also have permeated the creation of the EEA. The regulation which launched the Agency was approved just over a year after it was first proposed by Delors in a speech to the EP - a very short time in EC terms (CEC, 1990b). The only remaining detail was to find the EEA an institutional home, and all Member States were invited to submit candidate sites. At the time of the Council decision, the Commission 'confidently expected that a decision on the site (would) be made in the next few weeks' (CEC, 1990e, p. 1).

However, France continued to block the approval of a site for the EEA on the grounds that no new EC-related institutions should be sited until permanent homes are found for existing ones. The French wanted assurances that the EP would continue to hold its plenary sessions in Strasbourg despite mounting disenchantment throughout the EC about the EP's irrational housekeeping arrangements. (1) Ripa di Meana, as well as national environment ministers such as the UK's Michael Heseltine, launched blistering attacks on the French for holding the EEA's creation hostage to petty national interests (see Lambert and Wilkie, 1992).

In short, the development of EC preventive policies is hampered by a wide range of political disputes which are unrelated to the actual merits of new policies. The EC is often characterised as a generally technocratic system of policy making, but it has become more highly politicised as a policy making system since the mid-1980s, especially due to raging theological disputes about its future institutional development. These points are amply illustrated in the case studies of EC preventive policy making which follow.

IV. Case studies

Water quality

While the SEA significantly extended the EC's competence in environmental policy, recent controversies surrounding common water quality standards are rooted in directives passed in the 1970s. The 1976 EC Directive on Bathing Water Quality has been a key point of contention between the Commission and Member States, particularly the UK. As Ward's chapter indicates, many British seaside towns and cities continue to dump raw sewage into the sea close to beaches. Because this pollution tends to circulate away from the UK and toward the continent, Milne (1987) argues that incentives for the UK to discontinue the practice are weak.

The UK is by no means the only violator of EC rules. In 1990 the Commission began infraction proceedings against no fewer than 10 other Member States (Lewis, 1991, p. 63). The case of bathing water quality illustrates the degree to which the Commission depends on Member States to monitor their own compliance. Only Belgium, Luxembourg, and the UK correctly tested all of their beaches in 1989-90 (Schoon, 1991).

The British attitude toward EC rules, as summarised by a Department of the Environment (DoE) spokesman, is echoed throughout the Community: 'The [EC] standard for viruses is zero. You could reach that, but you'd have to shoot all the seagulls first' (quoted in Williams, 1991). What makes the UK unique among Member States is that its national legislation designed to comply with the EC directive has so few provisions for informing the public. For example, the DoE does not include virus test results in its published lists of beaches which meet EC standards, whereas French law requires that test results be displayed publicly (Lewis, 1991, p. 62).

A separate EC directive on drinking water quality was adopted in 1980. By 1989, most EC Member States still failed to meet its standards and the Commission began infringement proceedings against six Member States including the UK (Lewis, 1991, p. 67). The Commission admitted that the directive was adopted at a time when the state of knowledge about the harmfulness of water pollutants - especially pesticides -

was in its infancy. But DG XI officials were quick to note:

> [T]he pesticide parameter ... is not something which was decided by the Commission, but rather was decided by the Member States ... [It] was not even proposed by the Commission, but rather by a group of national experts which worked as part of the preparation of this Directive. These young people with high ambitions for the protection of the environment and health took the point of view that pesticides should be used in such a way that they did not find their way into drinking water ... Thus, there should be no doubt that the pesticide parameter in the Drinking Water Directive has to be seen in a political context (Henningsen, 1990,pp. 6-7).

Yet, national governments complain that the Commission wants more from them than is realistic or necessary. They find support from scientists (see North, 1989a; Wilkie, 1992) and the agrochemical industry, which argues that: 'the EC seem[s] to show a disturbing unawareness of the very significant amounts of good data which have been produced showing that the effects of pesticides ... are not really as great as had been assumed' (Foulkes, 1990, p. 118).

The case of water quality yields three key observations. First, it illustrates a problem shared by all public environmental protection agencies, but especially the EC. Choosing acceptable levels of pollution is a complex, technical and often arbitrary process. The actual enforcement of standards can become highly politicised. To illustrate the point, the Commission's case alleging unacceptable levels of nitrates in East Anglian drinking water in 1989 originally was compiled by Stanley Clinton Davis, a former Labour politician and Ripa di Meana's predecessor as Environment Commissioner. The Commission took its action at a time when its frustration with the Thatcher government's general irascibility on a range of EC issues had peaked. Meanwhile, British Ministers insisted that the UK enforced whatever it *did* agree to, in contrast to lax southern Member States. Water provided a perfect opportunity to expose the UK as ignoring regulations to which it previously had assented (see North, 1989b).

Second, environmental pressure groups work closely with the Commission. They are poised to exploit any opportunity to draw public attention to the degradation of the environment. The enhanced vigilance - even aggressiveness - of the Commission in recent years stems in part from the increase in the number of complaints it has received from private citizens and pressure groups about the application of EC standards. More than 465 complaints were lodged in 1989, up from 190 in 1988 and only 11 in 1985 (Lewis, 1991, p. 68). The Friends of the Earth submitted the original complaint about nitrates in East Anglian drinking water. The British Consumer Association generated considerable publicity in August 1991 by publishing its own tests of virus levels at the UK's 15 best-known beaches, which showed that all but one failed to meet EC standards (Williams, 1991).

Third, a puzzle emerges. The Commission has a mandate to hold governments to standards which appear over-strict and unrealistic, but ones to which Member States have agreed in past Council decisions. Part of the explanation is that governments often agree to try to meet tough standards over relatively long periods of time. When these periods are longer than electoral cycles (as they usually are), there is a tendency to accept over-ambitious proposals for acceptable standards because of the symbolic political capital to be gained in agreeing to them. Compliance is then ordinarily the responsibility of some future government.

In its enthusiasm for new preventive policies, the Commission often appears heedless of the costs or social implications of its campaigns to embarrass Member States into compliance with EC pollution laws. In the case of the bathing quality directive, even the Friends of the Earth acknowledged that the zero standard for viruses was unrealisable (Williams, 1991). However, the point is that ultimately it is EC governments themselves which determine the standards which the Commission is obligated to uphold.

Auto emissions

The setting of EC-wide auto emission standards for small cars in 1985 left a legacy of intense conflict between states, interest groups, and EC institutions. Member States with stronger environmental records (Denmark), domestic industries which specialise in 'big cars' (Germany) or no domestic auto industry at all (the Netherlands) preferred tight emission standards and a strict timetable for implementation.   Countries producing mainly small cars (Britain, France, Spain, Italy) argued that the costs of implementing stricter emission controls would render their products uncompetitive and benefit their Japanese competitors.

After substantial bickering and bargaining, the Council of Ministers agreed a new common position on 'clean cars' in 1988 which was designed to update the 1985 directive. The new position stipulated that after October 1993, new small cars would have to meet standards stricter than those embodied in the 1985 agreement, but not as strict as those in the US or Japan. The new package pleased nobody. Among Member States, a North-South divide emerged with the Netherlands, Denmark and Germany arguing that the proposed standards were not strict enough and feeble compared to tougher US and Canadian rules. Southern states led by France claimed that the new standards were too rigid. Britain's car industry also stood to suffer under the new proposal. UK manufacturers, more than any other Community producers, had invested heavily in the development of 'lean burn' technology which, although able to bring about a significant cut in emission levels, could not match the proposed norms.

The umbrella pressure group, the Liaison Committee of European Community Automobile Constructors (CLCA), joined the southern states in lobbying the Commission and EP against stricter norms. They claimed that the proposed norms would leave the industry in an uncertain and uncompetitive position. In particular, they argued that the fitting of three-way catalytic converters necessary to meet the emissions level could increase the cost of a new small car by 13-15 per cent.

A rival umbrella group, the European Environmental Bureau (EEB), complained that the Council's position was a 'revealing example of the inadequate character of the European strategy for environmental protection' (EIS, 1989a, p. 6). Speaking for more than 100 individual environmental groups, the EEB called on the Parliament to make use of its 'second reading' to force amendments to the Council's common position.

The EP eagerly took up the battle. It drastically amended the Council's common position, insisting that norms be obligatory from 1993 which were 'at least as strict' as US standards (quoted in *Financial Times*, 27 July 1990). The EP threatened that if its amendments were not accepted, it would reject outright the Council's position. Had the Parliament done so, the Council would have had to act unanimously (an unlikely prospect) to over-turn the EP's proposed amendments.

The Commission was forced to reassess its position. In April 1989, one week before the EP's threatened vote, the Commission announced that it was set to propose stricter small car emission standards (EIS, 1989a, p. 7). The issue then returned to the Council of Ministers, where the UK emerged as a hinge player in the North-South divide. Despite the British reservations about stricter norms, the UK faced domestic political constraints. The Thatcher government's abrupt conversion to environmentalism and a looming EP election clashed with the temptation to block an important anti-pollution agreement.

In June 1989, the stricter motion was passed by the Council, with only Greece and Denmark opposing it. (2) Environmentalists hailed the agreement as a case of environmental interests winning over the vested interests of small car producers and their home countries. The EP's Environment committee chairman, Ken Collins, boasted that, 'We forced the catalytic converter on a reluctant Britain and France,' (quoted in *The Independent*, 8 May 1990). David Grant Lawrence, a member of Ripa di Meana's cabinet, recalled: 'This was a turning point for the Commission. It came just before the European elections. It was becoming clear that the Greens would do well everywhere. No minister could afford to be seen to sabotage a good decision' (quoted in *The Independent*, 8 May 1990).

This case study illustrates the multidimensional nature of conflict surrounding preventive issues. The setting of new standards was marked by three distinct but overlapping dimensions of conflict: the struggle between Member States (i.e. France and Denmark); between pressure groups (i.e. the CLCA and EEB), and between EC institutions (i.e. the Parliament and Council). The result was an EC policy which set a minimum level of environmental protection which was higher than could have been achieved at a domestic level in most EC Member States.

Food hygiene

The Commission and EP have been at the forefront of EC efforts to harmonise disparate national health regulations and thus iron out many distortions to competition. In 1988, the EP requested that the Commission produce a draft directive on general food hygiene. The request urged that EC rules were needed to ensure that the same high standards applied to food manufacturers and retailers throughout the 12 Member States.

At an early stage of policy formation, the Commission must decide which DG is to produce draft legislation. For a directive on food hygiene, the candidates include the food division of DG III (Internal Market), DG VI (Agriculture) or DG XI (Environmental and Consumer Protection). In this case, instead of waiting for a Commission decision on jurisdiction, the Agricultural Directorate produced its own rule book and presented it to the EP for an Opinion. Incensed, DG III drew up a separate list of rules.

The EP issued a series of reports and oral questions to highlight the incoherence of the Commission's proposals. In her report on minced meat regulation, UK MEP Pauline Green complained that 'this is just another proposal in a long series of Regulations on specific food hygiene matters that the [Consumer Affairs] Committee has had to examine in the last 18 months ... It is often asked to express an Opinion on proposals from one DG while another DG is circulating quite a different draft' (quoted in EIS, 1991, p. 8). In response, the Commissioner for Agriculture, Ray MacSharry, warned that the EP had to avoid delays 'if the objectives of the internal market are to be achieved on schedule' (quoted in EIS, 1991, p. 8).

Diffuse patterns of policy making have consequences for implementation. A plethora of specific regulations - proposed by separate DGs - makes life more difficult for food manufacturers, consumers and control bodies. Competing regulations often imply different production standards, temperature rules and implementing arrangements, often for the same plant or distribution or retail network. For example, under the competing 1988 proposals a towel could be used several times by workers handling fresh meat but only once if they are handling meat pies. Freda Stack of the UK Co-op Union attacked the Commission for its lack of coordination and offered, 'Frankly, what they need is cabinet government' (quoted in *The Independent*, 5 May 1991).

Conflicts between Member States complicate the issue. For example, a draft regulation developed by the Commission in 1991 deemed that some cuts of meat - such as head, belly, and shin - should not be used in the manufacture of sausage. While the regulation was acceptable to most Member States, British manufacturers opposed it and insisted that these parts 'add to the flavour'.

The case of food hygiene offers a prime example of the complex political dynamics surrounding the making of EC preventive policy. Notable here are rivalries within the Commission and between the Commission and Parliament. As in other areas of preventive policy, decisions are often more political than practical as rival institutions seek to preserve and assert their powers. Moreover, this case illustrates the difficulties surrounding the implementation of EC regulations at the national level. Hapless firms are faced with haphazard and even contradictory EC rules because different regulations are made within discrete policy networks. In sum, the road from a good 'preventive' idea to a successful EC policy is normally a long one marked by multiple twists and perils.

Tobacco advertising and labelling

A key thrust of EC health policy since 1989 has been stricter regulation of tobacco product advertising and labelling. The Commission has justified its intervention on the grounds that patchwork national regulatory regimes give some manufacturers unfair advantages over others and thus violate the principle of the internal market. In September 1989, the Commission secured agreement from the Council of Health Ministers on a directive which banned tobacco advertising near schools and required that common health warnings be featured in advertisements and on cigarette packets. The new warnings included stark messages such as 'smoking kills.'

The directive was passed by majority vote despite British opposition. Afterwards, two years of negotiations between the British government and the tobacco industry were required before an agreement on implementing the EC directive could be secured. Even then, the agreement to carry the new health warnings and gradually eliminate advertising near schools was purely voluntary. It was criticised by the Secretary of the British Medical Association as: 'too limited to be effective and lack(ing) any urgency' (quoted in Hall, 1991).

In 1991, the directive was extended to cover all tobacco products, including pipe tobacco and cigars (EIU, 1991). At the same time, the Commission unveiled proposals for a total ban on the advertising of all tobacco products. Vasso Papandreou, the Social Affairs Commissioner, claimed that seven Member States supported the proposal, but admitted that others - including the UK and Germany - remained skeptical (quoted in *Agence Europe*, 12/13 November 1991, p. 11). The British in particular argued that the ban would threaten the continued viability of many sporting events - particularly auto and boat races - which depended on sponsorship by tobacco companies.

This case study highlights three key points. First, the British government continues to shun formalised regulatory arrangements as a method of achieving the goals set out in EC directives. The use of directives accommodates the peculiarly voluntaristic style of regulation in the UK. Agreements can take a long time to appear and compliance usually is left to industry itself.

A second point is that governments often use the EC as a leverage device for getting industry to conform to its wishes. It was widely reported that the UK Department of Health threatened to support the Commission's proposal to ban advertising altogether in 1991 unless the British tobacco industry finally agreed to adopt the new Euro-health warnings (see Hall, 1991). Governments will usually go to bat at the EC for their domestic industries, but this support is rarely unconditional. Public agencies often seek to empower themselves within domestic policy networks by threatening to simply accept stringent new EC laws when the behaviour of domestic industries embarrasses governments politically at the EC level.

Finally and more generally, the tobacco directives point to a new activism on the part of both the Commission and the EC Health Council in developing EC health policies which are genuinely preventive. The Council in 1991 directed the Commission to prepare reports on health policy and the single market and the relationship between health and the environment. It also sought an agreement on common measures to counter the doping of athletes before the 1992 Olympic games. The Maastricht treaty (if ratified) will give the EC new competence over the cross-border aspects of health. It reflects a broad consensus among Member States - leaving aside the UK - on the point that health policies should become more preventive in method, and that the EC has a key role to play in the process.

V. Conclusion

The EC is a complex setting for policy making. This chapter has shown that EC preventive strategies are the product of multidimensional conflict between competing pressure groups, institutions and national interests. Technocratic rationality motivates many EC preventive policies. Yet, what makes preventive policies most interesting -

and what distinguishes them from many 'core' EC internal market policies - is that, by nature, they are caught up in wider debates about how much power should be surrendered by Member States to the EC in the interest of the 'common European good'.

In some cases, the EC can stand behind the subsidiarity principle. For example, pollution control is by nature a transboundary problem. Moreover, the Commission and EP can claim that the EC is the logical level of government for making preventive policies because the time horizons of national governments are restricted by electoral considerations. EC institutions can afford to be more concerned with Europe's quality of life in the long-term and less concerned with economic growth or electoral politics in the short-term. EC social policy can be justified on the grounds that action must be taken now to deal with the long-term problem of the ageing of the European workforce. A shrinking pool of labour means future workers must be healthier, more productive and less at risk to accidents in the workplace if Europe is to remain a first-rank economic competitor beyond 2000.

But preventive policies also are pursued by the Commission and EP because of their symbolic political value. The Commission and EP both compete to identify themselves as institutions at the vanguard of a movement (partly self-created) to improve the quality of life in Europe and make European government more responsive to new social concerns and lifestyles. To some extent, their efforts have struck a chord with European citizens. Stronger public support exists for a common EC environmental policy than for any other EC activity. More than 80 per cent of EC citizens consistently express support for common-European rules on the environment (CEC, 1990d, p. 15). A cull of Eurobarometer surveys reveals that this question regularly evokes 'the strongest, most positive, and most unanimous reaction of any question posed on common European policies' (EIS, 1989b, p. 2).

The essays in this collection have stressed the importance of ideology as a determinant of whether preventive policies are embraced by government and whether they succeed or fail. In many ways, the EC is a uniquely technocratic system for policy making, but ideology matters here, too. The EC is a forum for the mediation of competing ideologies which make different assumptions about the proper role of the state in European life generally and the proper role of the EC in European government more specifically. The radical liberalism of the UK often clashes with the *etatisme* of France or the 'social market' orientation of Germany. More broadly, preventive policy making is permeated with a conflict between visions of the EC as either a club of sovereign nations or as an integrated federal system.

As a system for the mediation of government-industry relations, the EC differs significantly from British government. Mills' opening chapter argues that British government-industry relations are based upon trust, close understandings and a relative lack of public scrutiny over policies. There is no single 'EC style' of policy making. But the growing power of the EC in environmental and consumer regulation and the new opportunities for influence it provides to groups such as the Friends of the Earth or CECG means that relations between EC institutions and industries affected by preventive policies are based far more on mistrust than trust.

The 'close understandings' which characterise British government-industry relations are precluded by the EC's complexity and the openness of most EC preventive policy networks to a vast range of interests. It is no easy matter for affected industrial groups to work out how the EC's policy making labyrinth operates. Once they do, the task of trying to locate and consolidate a winning coalition which will support their agenda is difficult and laborious.

As in British government, there is little public scrutiny of how EC policies are made, particularly at the level of the Council of Ministers, which is highly secretive and cliquish. However, the Commission and the EP are quite open and accessible to outside interests. Both must practice *engrenage* (Coombes, 1970, pp. 86-91) - or the intermeshing of all relevant interests - so that policy proposals are more likely to be accepted by the Council. The EC is by no means a Jeffersonian system of pluralism, but it often does provide newly organised interest groups with opportunities to side-step insular national policy networks which are impermeable by all but the most established interests.

Engrenage turns the argument about the EC's lack of democratic accountability on its head. To ensure a high quality of life, Europe clearly requires some policies that are technocratically-derived and politically costly to national governments. Sometimes, as shown in the cases of auto emissions or tobacco labelling, the EC's system works. The EC allows national governments to foist the blame onto Brussels for policies which threaten entrenched interests, such as auto or tobacco manufacturers. Europe gets cleaner air or water, less youths who smoke cigarettes, or fewer accidents in the workplace in the process. The logic of *engrenage* is that the Commission and EP can enhance the EC's credibility when they can demonstrate to Member States that EC policies contain tangible benefits for the 12 as a collective, while still leaving all relevant interests at least '51 per cent' satisfied.

The EC as a political system is still in the process of being constructed. Yet, any scenario which imagines the establishment of prevention as a central strategy in the making of a wide range of public policies ignores the fact that the EC is and will remain primarily a forum for policy formulation, not implementation. The debates on subsidiarity which consumed the EC in 1992 led to new interest in a 'Europe of the Regions', or a revamped policy process in which sub-national governments - which are often responsible for implementing EC policies 'on the ground' - play a greater role in decision making. However, as presently constituted, the EC's policy making process often fails to yield effective policies because both the Commission and EP as well as EC Member States are motivated their own political goals as much as effective and desirable policy outcomes.

The Commission and EP both have farsighted, even altruistic aims related to preventive policies. These aims sometimes dovetail neatly with their blatantly political agendas to expand their powers, but the continued expansion of the EC's role in preventive policy sectors is likely to occur only in fits and starts. The EC's institutions, like all other interests in EC politics, must accept that the politics of the EC is the politics of bargaining, compromise and incrementalism.

Footnotes

1) The EP meets as a whole in Strasbourg, its administration is based in Luxembourg, and its committees meet in Brussels.

2) The Greek position was that financial incentives should be employed instead of standards, while the Danes viewed the new norms as not strict enough.

Bibliography/references

Anderson, Christopher (1991), 'EC putting bite in its green bark', *New Scientist*, 18 July, p.182.

Bomberg, Elizabeth (1992), 'The German Greens and the European Community', *Environmental Politics*, December, vol. 1, no. 4, pp. 160-185.

Boons, Frank (1991), 'Environmental policy and the chemical industry in Europe: conflict, cooperation, and commercialization', paper presented at ECPR Joint Session of Workshops, Colchester, England, 22-8 March.

Bradshaw, Jeremy (1991), 'Institutional reform in the European Community beyond Maastricht', *European Trends*, The Economist Intelligence Unit, vol. 4, pp. 82-93.

Brinkhorst, Laurens (1991), 'Environment policy and the European Community', *Town and Country Planning*, January, pp. 18-21.

Butterworths European Information Services (1989), *Butterworths Guide to the European Communities* (including full Text of Treaty of Rome), Butterworths, London.

CEC (1990a), Common position on Environmental Research and Development for 1990-1994: Scientific and Technical Objectives and Content of the Programme, Commission of the European Communities, Brussels, COM 10897/1/90, Annex I.

CEC (1990b), 'Council regulation on the establishment of the European Environment Agency and the European Environment Information and Observation Network', *Official Journal of the European Communities*, vol. L 120, Commission of the European Communities, Brussels, EEC no. 1210/90, pp. 1-6.

CEC (1990c), *EC Research Funding: A Guide for Applicants*, Commission of the European Communities, Brussels.

CEC (1990d), *Environmental Policy in the European Community*, Commission of the European Communities, Luxembourg, 4th edition.

CEC (1990e), 'The European Environment Agency (EEA)', *DG XI Information Sheets*, Commission of the European Communities/DG XI, Brussels.

CEC (1990f), 'Socio-Economic Environmental Research (SEER): Part 3 of the environmental research programme 1990-94', Commission of the European Communities/DG XII-E, Brussels, third draft.

Clement, Barrie (1991), 'MPs dismiss EC social charter as "mirage"', *The Independent*, 21 August, p. 10.

Coombes, David (1970), *Politics and Bureaucracy in the European Community: A Portrait of the Commission of the E.E.C.*, George Allen and Unwin, London.

Corbett, Richard (1987), 'The 1985 Intergovernmental Conference and the Single European Act', in, Pryce, Roy (ed.), *The Dynamics of European Union*, Croom Helm, London, pp. 238-72.

Council of the European Communities and CEC (1992), 'Treaty on European Union',

Luxembourg, Office for the Official Publications of the European Communities.

Crampton, Stephen, and Judith Eversley (1990), 'People's Europe: a consumer viewpoint', *European Trends*, Economist Intelligence Unit, vol. 2, pp. 77-82.

Duff, A. N. (1986), 'Eureka and the new technology policy of the European Community',*Policy Studies*, vol. 6, April, pp. 44-61.

The Economist (1991a),'The strain of Spain', 27 April, p. 56.

The Economist (1991b), 'The dirty dozen', 20 July, p. 54.

EIS (1989a), 'Car pollution: Commission assures Parliament it will propose strict emission norms,' *European Environment Fortnightly*, European Information Service, Brussels, no. 319, 18 April, pp. 6-7.

EIS (1989b), 'Eurobarometer: strong support for common environmental protection measures,' *European Environment Fortnightly*, European Information Service, Brussels, no. 321, 23 May, p. 2.

EIS (1991), 'Food hygiene: Commission urges protection of internal market programme and Parliament calls for proposal on food hygiene', *European Environment Fortnightly*, European Information Service, Brussels, no. 363, 23 April, pp. 8-10.

EIU (1991), 'Tobacco labelling: sectoral report,' *European Trends*, Economist Intelligence Unit, vol. 4, p. 12.

EP (1990), Economic and fiscal incentives as a means of achieving environmental policy objectives, European Parliament Directorate-General for Research, Luxembourg, (Research and Documentation Paper - Environment, Public Health and Consumer Protection Series).

Foulkes, D. M. (1990), 'Symposium Review', in, Thomas, B. (ed), *Future Changes in Pesticide Registration within the EC*, British Crop Protection Council, Farnham, Surrey, proceedings of a Symposium held at the University of Reading, UK, 3-5 January 1990, BCPC monograph no. 44, pp. 117-21.

Freestone, David (1991), 'European Community environmental policy and law', *Journal of Law and Society*, vol. 18, Spring, pp. 135-54.

Hall, Celia (1991), 'New tobacco advertising agreement under attack', *The Independent*, 10 September, p. 6.

Henningsen, J. (1990), 'European Commission Objectives and the Single European Act,' in, Thomas, B. (ed), *Future Changes in Pesticide Registration within the EC*, British Crop Protection Council, Farnham, Surrey, (proceedings of a Symposium held at the University of Reading, UK, 3-5 January 1990), BCPC monograph no. 44, pp. 1-10.

Johnson, Stanley P., and Guy Corcelle (1989), *The Environmental Policy of the European Communities*, Graham and Trotman, London (International and Environmental Law and Policy Series).

Lambert, Sarah, and Tom Wilkie (1992), 'British tap water fails to meet EC standards,' *The Independent*, 22 January, p. 1.

Lewis, Claire Simone (1991), 'Application of environmental legislation in EC Member States: The bathing water and drinking water directives', *European Trends*, The Economist Intelligence Unit, vol. 4, pp. 59-68. .

Liberatore, Angela (1991), 'Problems of transnational policymaking: environmental policy in the European Community', *European Journal of Political Research*, vol. 19, March/April, pp. 281-305.

MacKenzie, Debora (1991a), 'Ministers clash over rules for modified organisms,' *New Scientist*, 3 August, p. 8.

Mackenzie, Debora (1991b), 'Fund to green Europe's poorer nations', *New Scientist*, 21 December, p. 6.

Marsh, David, and R. A. W. Rhodes (eds.) (1992), *Policy Networks in British Government*, Clarendon Press, Oxford.

Milne, R. (1987), 'Pollution and politics in the North Sea', *New Scientist*, 19 December, pp. 53-8.

North, Richard (1989a) 'Scientist defends standards of Britain's drinking water', *The Independent*, 22 September, p. 6.

North, Richard (1989b), 'Six factors that led to the EC prosecution', *The Independent*, 22 September, p. 6.

Peters, B. Guy (1992), 'Bureaucratic Politics and the Institutions of the European Community', in, Sbragia, Alberta M. (ed.), *Euro-Politics: Institutions and Policymaking in the 'New' European Community*, Brookings Institution, Washington, D.C., pp. 75-122.

Peterson, John (1989), 'Hormones, heifers and high politics: biotechnology and the Common Agricultural Policy', *Public Administration*, vol. 67, no. 4, Winter, pp. 455-71.

Peterson, John (1991), 'Technology policy in Europe: explaining the Framework programme and Eureka in theory and practice', *Journal of Common Market Studies*, vol. 29, no. 3, March, pp. 269-90.

Rhodes, Martin (1991), 'The social dimension of the Single European Market versus transnational regulation', *European Journal of Political Research*, vol.19, March/April, pp.245-80.

Schoon, Nicholas (1991), 'Low ratings for British beaches may be unfair,' *The Independent*, 10 September, p. 5.

Wilkie, Tom (1992), 'Scientists query logic of EC water purity standards', *The Independent*, 22 January, p. 3.

Williams, Rhys (1991), 'Beaches "fail to meet EC standards on viruses"', *The Independent*, 14 August, p. 3.

10   Liberalism, democracy and prevention

Mike Mills and Michael Saward

Of the various themes which run through the case studies in this volume, one of the most fundamental to explaining policy is the role of ideology. (1) The boundaries and styles of policy on prevention are, it seems, determined to a considerable degree by assorted values and assumptions concerning relationships between individuals, groups and the state. In Britain, these values and assumptions derive for the most part from the most basic operating principles of the political system, namely those principles bound up in the idea of liberal democracy.

In this chapter, we aim to explore the role of liberal democratic ideology in the field of preventive medicine. After examining those aspects of the case studies which reveal something of the roles which ideology plays, we step back to take a broader view of the ideas of liberty, liberalism and democracy. The core of the discussion will focus on the notions of negative and positive liberty, and the extent to which our case studies reveal that one or other basic interpretation of liberty has been dominant in this field of policy. Finally, we note some ways in which the idea of democracy can add weight to a particular interpretation of liberty, and in turn how this may provide a contrast with what we have learned about the understanding of liberty held by many of the relevant British government actors.

The cases revisited

Almost all of the case studies give some insight into the ways in which policy in this field is ideologically-driven. Taken together they make an argument for regarding ideology as a key explanatory variable in prevention policy. We should begin, therefore, by reminding ourselves of these insights.

Read's study of smoking offers very clear evidence of the central role of ideology. It involves not only the question of the right of the individual to choose (or, perhaps, to define and act upon their own interests as they see fit), but also the right of producers to produce and to make profits. This case raises many key questions about liberal democracy: just what is the responsibility of the state in such cases? Is it to protect peoples' health, or to support the wealth creation process? If there is to be a trade-off between these two values, then on the basis of what principle (or principles) can the trade-off be conducted?

Read's second case study, dealing with seat belts, raises some of these questions again, though it is perhaps more straightforward since government regulation in this field has far fewer commercial implications because it does not threaten the viability of the industry concerned. What is particularly interesting about the case of seat belts is the way that Parliament offers a forum for an often overt expression of ideology which is more often implicit in much of what the British state actually does. The debate between the 'individualists' and the 'collectivists' - and the ultimate success of the latter - belies the fact that much preventive policy is predicated upon very individualist assumptions.

Hann's study of breast cancer highlighted in particular how electoral short-termism can act as an important determinant of policy in a liberal democracy but also how values within professions can affect decision making and advice. Street's chapter on AIDS policy raises issues about the basis upon which the state might act to protect peoples' health. Here, it seems clear that the state makes its choices about which groups in society to protect on an ideological basis, as opposed to some more objective or rational (or liberal democratic?) basis. It is clear from the case of AIDS, therefore, that while health may be perceived as a public good, it has had to compete with values such as those regarding law and order, the family and sexuality which are very difficult to budge in a political sense.

Ward's chapter highlights a different dimension of the role of ideology, that of how evidence of health problems ought to be interpreted. Interpretation always takes place within a framework, and there is often no easy basis upon which to distinguish the proper framework to employ. Ward also draws our attention to the symbolic value of water as a cultural expression of social fears and prejudices which, in turn, qualifies the actions of government.

Lane's chapter on home births brings in ideology as an explanatory variable in two ways, namely the bureaucratic and technological controls women can be subject to, and the patriarchal assumptions which apparently inform state and professional activity in this area of policy. Lane's argument supports Read's assertion that ideology can have an institutional expression - in this case the concentration of birthing in hospitals rather than in the home. But it also draws our attention to the relationship between professionalisation, patriarchy and ideology; in short, it is not possible to explain why there are so few home births in Britain without appreciating that patriarchy exists.

Bomberg and Peterson's chapter on the EC acts, in some ways, as a control for the notion that ideology is important in the institutional sense. They argued that there is not a dominant ideological position within the institutions of the EC, which clearly offers a contrast to many of the other cases we have. As far as electoral short-termism was concerned, this made a significant difference to the adoption of preventive health policies, but it was also evident that Member States did have common interests as far as 'macro-controversies' were concerned, despite the fact that they disagreed on the balance that should be struck between, for example, individualist and collectivist approaches, the interventionism of the EC itself and their willingness to incur economic costs for the sake of preventive policies. However, they recognise that cross-national ideological differences do play a part in the formulation of policy and in the compromises which are eventually reached.

Allsop and Freeman also touch on the role of ideology through their consideration of the relationship between government and producer interests and also through their references to the professional arguments and cleavages which have accompanied the development of preventive policies over the past twenty years or so. Here we see that the values which a particular group represents does make a difference to their effect on public policy.

In sum, we would argue that six points appear to arise with regard to the role of (liberal democratic) ideology in prevention. These are:

(1) Should individuals be free to choose their own lifestyles? If they should be free in some cases and not others, then what is the dividing line?

(2) Should the state try to engineer or manipulate systemic or community influences on peoples' health, or rather point out to individuals what some of those influences are?

(3) On what bases has the state decided which groups or individuals should be helped? Should the criterion be vulnerability, or responsibility, or what?

(4) To what extent is patriarchy a limiting or constraining influence?

(5) How does the state reconcile the rights of the individual with the relatively free operation of the market?

(6) To what extent does the role of ideology filter even into the area of the use and interpretation of empirical evidence?

With these points isolated and made explicit, we shall now move on to consider some of the key tensions involved in the effort to resolve these issues. Our aim is not to make large moral claims, but rather to elucidate as fully as possible in the available space the character of the ideological questions that have been raised.

Liberty and Liberalism

On one view, the key points about ideology arising from the case studies are disparate. However, we would argue that they all involve basic issues about the relationships between individuals, the market and the state. As such, they connect very closely with some of the core questions of liberalism, and in particular its conception of liberty for individuals and groups. We need, then, to take a closer look at the ideology of liberalism. In many respects, the most important question to be addressed is 'what is the proper focus and extent of state activity?' When this question is asked, the most basic distinction - or tension within the ideology of liberalism - comes to the fore: should liberty be conceived as positive liberty or negative liberty?

In some of the case studies in this volume, this has been clear in terms of some of the ways in which individual liberty has been invoked as an obstacle to certain preventive health policies (e.g. seat belts and smoking). To a degree, liberalism's account of liberty is most relevant to 'individual' preventive strategies, as opposed to community and systemic strategies (see Mills's chapter above), since it is concerned with efforts to alter the behaviour of individuals. However, this three part distinction is more of a practical, and not a substantive, distinction. It concerns strategies appropriate to the scale and type of the problems faced, rather than the end desired. Hence, the categories overlap considerably when it comes to the nature of the problem itself, and to the role of the state. When systemic strategies are preferred, in general, we can say that we are normally dealing with cases where some plausible combination of (a) the number of people harmed, and (b) the extent of the harm caused is very high as well as involuntarily assumed (such as with the greenhouse effect). Thus, we will have to deal also with liberalism's account of large scale harms which are not questions of individual choice in the first instance. In particular, such cases often involve corporations, property rights and the quality of the external environment in a liberal society. We shall deal with these below.

There are two quite different stories told by liberals which have direct relevance to preventable harms which are, in the first instance, products of individual choice. The clearest way to distinguish between them is to invoke Berlin's famous distinction between negative and positive freedom (or liberty). (2) The version of liberalism which defines liberty in terms of negative freedom stresses the point that a person is free if there is an absence of restraint (Plant, 1991, p. 221) - someone is 'free from' something. Restraint here is seen for the most part as state interference in the choices that individuals can make on the basis of their own desires and preferences. In other words, individuals, to be free, are seen as 'free from' outside interference in their choices.

Positive freedom, on the other hand, sees liberty as linked to a person's capacity to act to realise their goals in life - someone is 'free to' do something. This might be construed in a number of ways. For example, a writer in the positive freedom tradition might pinpoint what they regard as certain key interests or needs of individuals which are crucial for that person being truly free; or perhaps single out certain basic resources (like money or minimal property holdings) that a person would need in order to be able to take advantage of their negative liberty. Some accounts broadly accept the 'negative liberty' definition but focus on the value of liberty. That is, someone might be negatively free, as it were, but be so bereft of basic resources that that negative freedom has no real value for them, since they are not in a position to take advantage of it (Plant, 1991; Rawls, 1971).

In terms of preventive health policy, an advocate of the negative freedom approach would stress the fact that the decision (for example, whether or not to smoke, or whether or not to wear seat belts), is rightly one for each individual to make as he or she sees fit. The only point of any real importance to such an analyst is whether or not the state is interfering in the making of that choice. On this account, there is very little scope to discuss positive state action to prevent preventable harms to individuals.

Negative libertarians do allow for a 'minimal state', generally speaking.   This minimal state can exist to provide and enforce the necessary legal framework for market exchanges, and to provide certain 'indivisible' public goods, such as defence (see Nozick 1974, for example).   This is to say little more than that negative libertarians are not on the whole anarchists; they do see some role for the state, though not one that extends beyond a small range of more or less unavoidable functions, which may also include dealing with some risks that individuals cannot choose to avoid. Beyond this, what is good for each person can and should be decided by each and every person for themselves. If an individual voluntarily assumes a risk, then that is their business and right, and theirs alone.

An account from positive freedom, on the other hand, would stress the point that certain individuals may need help to take advantage of the absence of state restraint. It might emphasise, for example, the point that each individual in a society has a fundamental interest in preserving their health, so far as is reasonably possible. Without this, it might be argued, the absence of constraint - by the state or by other groups or individuals - will mean very little to many individuals.   A person's health is inextricably tied up with their capacity to realise whatever particular life plan they may have. A state which does not act in certain ways to minimise certain preventable risks, especially if they are not voluntarily assumed and often even if they are to some degree, is actually choosing not to optimise the sum total of freedoms experienced by its subject population. Thus, on the positive view, liberalism in its account of liberty can be taken to involve a variety of forms of state activity to (for instance) accurately inform citizens of the consequences of certain risks or even to place barriers in the way of possible individual actions that may be deleterious to an individual's health.

The distinction between negative and positive liberty has formed a fault line down the middle of liberal thought for many decades. It is also intimately connected to conceptions of rights within liberal ideology. The key liberal thinkers of modern times can be seen, in broad terms, to line up of different sides of this debate. Rawls, for example, is clearly in the positive liberty camp given (a) his concerns for what may be required for the absence of restraint to be meaningful for an individual; and (b) in his account of primary goods in *A Theory of Justice* (1971). Hayek and Nozick, in different ways, line up clearly on the side of negative freedom, stressing variously its relative simplicity (since apparently it does not involve discussion of interests, abilities, power or resources) and the fact that (supposedly) it does not 'moralise' the notion of freedom, since it says nothing about what private choices people ought to make (see Plant, 1991).

The basic schism at the heart of liberalism is familiar enough. Williams for instance has observed that: 'we find liberalism in the modern period dividing into at least two powerful perspectives, both of which use the vocabulary of "the individual" and "freedom", but one of which embraces state intervention while the other rejects it' (1991, p. 157). He goes on to observe that: 'liberalism cannot be seen as an aggregate of its various elements, because these elements are often in tension if not in conflict ... Nothing can collapse these rival conceptions of freedom and their political implications into a single essence ... ' (1991, p. 157, 158).

So, in many of the cases here the problem of how much state intervention there should be, and in whose interests it should work, can be seen as problems which are at the very heart of liberalism and which present governments with a classic liberal dilemma.

It remains in this section for us to focus on what liberalism's account of liberty might have to say on the question of systemic, or large scale, comprehensive and normally involuntary (for any one individual) harms caused to whole communities by one event or process. The paradigm case of such harms today is the impact of large corporations on the external environment, and therefore on the basic living conditions, of citizens. In terms of harms that were more to do with individual behaviour, we found an irreducible schism between two approaches to liberty. Does liberalism have anything clearer to say with regard to this slightly different area of risks and harms?

Liberalism's heyday was in the eighteenth and nineteenth centuries, an era devoid of strong or systematic state intervention into citizens' economic and social affairs. (3) As a result of this, the story told by the likes of Locke, Jefferson and Bentham was very much in line with what we now call negative liberty. In Locke's and Jefferson's cases, the rights of individuals not to have their liberties interfered with by government was stressed. What this came down to, most often, was that individual property rights could not be turned over by the state. Thus, on this Lockean view, oneself and one's possessions were equally one's own business. This included anyone's right to control and use their property as they saw fit within a permissive minimal legal framework.

This Lockean view was prominent at a time when relatively small property holdings were regarded as a key factor in political and social equality. Over time, however, with the development of corporate capitalism, liberal rights to property have become a justification for large scale inequalities between citizens. As Dahl has written: ' ... the agrarian socioeconomic order was destined to be wholly superseded by corporate capitalism. And as an unregulated external force, corporate capitalism would automatically generate acute inequalities in the distribution of property as well as other social and economic resources' (1985, p. 72). 'Thus', Dahl goes on, 'an economic order that spontaneously produced inequality in the distribution of economic and political resources acquired legitimacy, at least in part, by clothing itself in the recut garments of an outmoded ideology in which private ownership was justified on the ground that a wide diffusion of property would support political equality' (1985, p. 73).

Broader socio-economic inequalities affect the likelihood of the individual approach to prevention being successful for certain classes of the population, and they also make the voice of those who are politically and economically disadvantaged that much more difficult to hear. While it would be an overstatement to argue that all inequalities, and their effects on prevention, can be put down to the inherent problems of the defence of property rights, nevertheless, it is not difficult to see how the emphasis on individualism and property as the primary source of political equality, as found in certain versions of negative liberty, can and does leave other salient inequalities under represented on political agendas.

For our present purposes we can regard 'health' in general as one of Dahl's 'other social and economic resources'. Large scale threats to the health of large segments of the population were posed by these new political and economic developments. Furthermore, these were threats, like pollution of various kinds, which those subject to them could have little (if any) control over. The set of considerations here would appear to be different in kind from those considered above in terms of individual liberty and behaviour - mostly because of their sheer scale. The positive and negative views of freedom for individuals were irreconcilable: but is there more internal consistency within liberal ideology when it comes to this qualitatively and quantitatively different class of concerns?

The answer is, if anything, that liberals are likely to be almost just as strongly divided when it comes to these large scale concerns. The extent of the divisions between positive and negative freedom here may not be quite so great as for individual cases because negative libertarians are not opposed to state activity *tout court*, as noted briefly above. Beyond the provision of minimal legal frameworks, they will often be prepared to concede a role for the state if, for example, (a) only the state can make a difference in a certain case, or (b) where state activity or intervention today can free up the range of market choices available to individuals tomorrow (the theory, if not the actuality, of council house sales and opt-out schools in recent years in Britain).

For the positive libertarian, on the other hand, the response if anything is likely to be in favour of even stronger state action than in cases primarily involving individual choice. This is so because, having already accepted one of the paradigmatic arguments for state intervention in more 'individual' cases (see above), the intellectual tools exist to extend this intervention when the potentially deleterious effects on citizens' health, from certain industrial processes for example, grow. Thus, while the position of the negative libertarian would be little changed, that of the positive libertarian - perceiving, for example, that the value of negative freedom was diminishing all the more in systemic cases - moves further away still, toward stronger state intervention. On the face of it, the basic divisions between the two versions of liberty within liberalism seem to be just as far apart as they were with regard to individual harms.

Conceivably, negative libertarians might come close to agreeing on the morally permissable levels of state intervention (beyond the limited state already mentioned) if the state itself was centrally involved in the creation or provocation of a systemic harm to citizens. Thus, if a nationalised industry polluted water supplies in a residential area, on a basic principle of responsibility a negative libertarian might agree that the state should intervene to reverse its deleterious effects on the private lives of citizens. This principle of responsibility may arise for state enterprises because the state has, in principle, no business being *in* that business in the first place. The principle would not apply to private enterprises.

This has necessarily been a highly truncated discussion of liberalism and liberty, but nevertheless some key points have emerged. We looked to the ideology of liberalism to see if some relatively clear prescription was evident which might guide our thoughts on preventive health policies. What we have found is an apparently irreparable fault line. The nature and value of liberty for individuals can plausibly be construed in two basic ways; and these ways constitute nearly polar opposite points of view in terms of policy prescription. This was true, however, in different ways (and to different extents) for harms that are (a) primarily individual and voluntarily assumed, and (b) harms that are more systemic or environmental (and involuntarily assumed) in nature. In other words, we have found not one story, but at least two.

What is more, within liberalism there seem to be few theoretical resources to adjudicate between the two stories. That is, at the heart of liberalism there is a scepticism about the nature of the good life - or at least about any detailed or substantial account of it. What is good for one person, beyond a handful of basic facilitative legal provisions, may not be good for the next, and so on: the liberal will not intervene into this or that person's choice. This scepticism is in part a denial of foundations within liberalism - metaphysical foundations, as it were - which might otherwise be appealed to as a guide to sorting out more surface level clashes between prescriptions. There is no higher level principle which, within liberalism, we can appeal to in order to try to reconcile the competing wings of the ideology (see Goodin, 1988, for an example of an attempt to appeal to such a principle).

Many of the key points about ideology to emerge from the case studies help to illustrate the basic tensions within liberal ideology between negative and positive conceptions of liberty. In a sense, the liberal democratic state is caught somewhere between the two conceptions. This may be an overarching reason for its apparently inconsistent approach to prevention in different areas. It moves to promote health actively in some areas and is seemingly reluctant to act - or acts half-heartedly - in others. Perhaps the key point to note is that liberalism, and what it has to say about liberty, leaves plenty of room for interpretation at the level of policy. Liberalism as an ideology is not policy-specific; consistency between cases cannot be expected because the principles that are relevant are necessarily interpreted by policy makers.

Of course, on one level, this makes liberalism very difficult to use as part of our explanation for the (in)consistency of preventive policies because the same type of ideological issue, say the freedom of the individual, could have two different political responses (see, for example, those of seat belts and smoking). On another level, however, it is more useful because it points us towards the consistency with which liberal values have been applied across our case studies, even if the eventual policy outcome cannot be explained in terms of those values alone. Liberal values clearly have acted as constraints on policy even if they have met with a variable degree of success. Under this type of constraint it would not be unreasonable to expect that health problems which some may define as self-inflicted, AIDS or smoking-related illness, might find less favour with the state than the protection of those groups which have historically been seen as vulnerable through no fault of their own - e.g. women and children. This is not to say that these conceptions of the 'worthiness' of groups are correct, but rather, to point out that liberalism does have a problem in deciding when, and for whose benefit, the state should become active.

Democracy

By definition, liberal democracy does not just involve ideas about individual and corporate liberty. Liberal democracy is liberalism tempered and modified by the logic of democracy (see Beetham, 1992). In our view, by examining the democratic side of the liberal democratic equation we can take the above discussion further. Specifically, certain basic tenets at the heart of the idea of democracy help us to clarify the basic tension identified at the heart of liberalism.

Democracy is standardly defined as meaning 'rule of the people'. The notions of rule and people are radically unclear, and in the literature on democratic theory much space is devoted to their explication (see for example Held, 1987; Lively, 1975;

May, 1978). For our purposes, what is more important than entering into this semantic debate is to notice how democracy differs from liberalism. Liberalism - whether in its positive freedom or negative freedom guise - starts with ideas about individuals, their rights and their liberties. Anything more than a minimal, contract-enforcing role for the state in the lives of individual citizens has to be justified separately, though this will be done in different ways by different liberal theorists, politicians and bureaucrats. Democracy, by contrast, starts with a notion of *government*: in the general definition, somebody, *the people*, rules. Democracy 'is not a way of life but a form of government' (Parekh, 1992, p. 165). Ruling, governing, the sovereignty of one group of people over another - these things are implied in the term 'democracy'. Perhaps democracy can even be seen as a second order notion, with little to say on abstract philosophical questions, whereas liberalism includes a range of first order claims. As a result, democracy has less to say about natural or pre-social individual autonomy.

A good deal can be said about what it means to believe in democracy. To begin with, democracy is about the state being responsive to citizen demands, and hence liable to be activist and interventionist if that is what most people want. Further, and equally importantly, if one professes democracy, then presumably one believes that democratic systems ought to persist after their founding. Presumably also, then, one would wish to see enshrined those constitutional and other provisions which make up the logically necessary preconditions of democracy. This set of concerns has been expressed in terms of the 'self-binding' (Salecl, 1991; Elster, 1988) of democracy, and has clear resonances with (for example) Rawls's (1971) ('positive') discussion of liberty only rightly being restricted in the name of liberty itself.

We use the term 'constitutional and other provisions' that are necessary to limit democracy in order to protect it (e.g. to prevent a majority voting to abolish democratic institutions). Constitutional provisions in a democracy must include standard 'liberal' freedoms - of speech, association and information - and rights to (for example) vote unimpeded and uncoerced and to equal status of citizenship. These provisions are akin to the liberal notion of negative freedom, as discussed above.

'Other provisions' are, however, logically necessary for democracy to endure. In particular, if voting (nationally and in other contexts) is the paradigmatic form of preference registration (though not of preference formation) in a democracy, then certain provisions are logically necessary to render the vote - and its casting by any one citizen - meaningful. We would like to single out two such provisions which are often neglected in the broader literature on democratic thought: literacy and physical mobility.

For a citizens' registration of preference - a formal act - to be meaningful, he or she must have achieved a certain minimal level of literacy: that is, be able to read, write and comprehend the material produced by political parties and other commentators. Equally, he or she must have basic physical mobility, in the first instance in order to be able to get to the polls, but more generally to be able to have ready contact with other citizens to take part in the process of preference formation without unavoidable restraint. Clearly, there are many other, probably more powerful arguments, in favour of (for instance) paying more attention to the physical mobility of the physically handicapped. For the moment, however, it is the more or less instrumental considerations that are internal to democratic argument that concern us.

In terms of preventive health policy, the implications of such provision can be enormous. If a government is democratically chosen, and it professes democracy, then by logic it must perform certain actions, or pursue certain policies, to protect the democratic rights of citizens, beyond the basic task of being responsive to citizen demands. Briefly put, if a government can act to protect (for example) those aspects of a citizen's health which are vital for (to continue the example) basic physical mobility, then it has a democratic obligation to do so; conversely, citizens have a democratic right to such protections in principle. In a sense, because democracy is about 'government', and not (as with liberalism) first order concerns about the nature of 'individuals', it includes both 'positive' and 'negative' elements. The main difference between the ideologies of democracy and liberalism in this area is that the internal logic of democracy gives us a way of separating and sorting state actions into negative and positive categories.

We can see, then, that the idea and practice of democracy tempers liberalism when we speak of liberal democracy. It does so in two related ways. First, the idea of democracy suggests a necessary correspondence between citizen demands and state actions. If a majority of citizens demand strong state activity to prevent or alleviate certain risks to the health of citizens, then these are demands that a liberal democratic state should find it hard to resist in practice. Second, the very notion of democracy implies that individual citizens have democratic rights which the state is obliged to protect. These rights will include at least some of the major concerns in the area of prevention and health. The upshot of all this is that the idea of positive liberty is reinforced by the idea of democracy; and hence, in a liberal democratic political system, the weight of the arguments suggests a positive, active state rather than a negative, minimal state.

Of course, politics, especially in a democracy, is a messy business. Governments have many, often conflicting pressures placed upon them. In addition, there are many, often competing principles which governments might use to guide the shaping and implementing of public policy. Acting democratically may, and often will, be tempered by the demands of stability, efficiency, and so on. Saying how trade-offs between competing principles ought to be sorted out - if indeed they can be at all on some reasonable basis - is outside the scope of this chapter. The important point for present purposes is that we have, within the logic of democracy, identified a space for preventive health policy.

We must now return to some of the main points on ideology in the case studies in the light of the above discussion.

Conclusion: the case studies and ideology

The case studies, as noted above, often demonstrate the state's reluctance to adopt policy stances akin to positive liberty. Rather, they demonstrate that, if anything, the state tends to adopt a negative libertarian stance (on smoking, for example). We would argue that this sort of approach to prevention by the state is evident in the six points arising from the cases stated at the beginning of this chapter. Specifically, a slant towards a negative libertarian stance helps to explain, in general terms, the role of ideology in helping to explain the outcomes of public policy. (4)

The idea that individuals should be autonomous with regard to life choices was seen as an explanation for government action on smoking, seat belts and AIDS. On the subject of homebirths, it was argued that what is needed is an assertion or strengthening of individual autonomy, and a lessening of technological, male control over women's reproductive functions.   This ambiguity - liberalism's notion of autonomy seen as both friend and foe, as it were - ought not be surprising. It is a product of the deep ambiguities at the heart of liberal ideology itself. Liberalism, in its conception of liberty, offers no clear guidance on the question of the role of the state and the role of the citizen in such areas. We would suggest, however, that the idea of autonomy is more meaningful within the logic of democracy. To be able to form and express their preferences, citizens in a democracy need physical mobility: this is a core part of their capacity to express themselves without requiring more aid from others than may be absolutely necessary. This is a basic democratic right. The degree of immediacy, and the extent, of the threats to citizen's health of car accidents where seat belts are not worn, smoking and contracting the AIDS virus will differ; the democratic right to at least minimal protection from these risks is, however, clear enough. Thus, action in such cases which is directed to enhancing physical mobility, and therefore to enhancing autonomy, can be justified and explained in democratic terms. Seen this way, the accounts of seat belts, smoking and AIDS fall into line with demands for democratic autonomy with respect to homebirths, and it is the democratic, as much as the liberal, aspects of liberal democracy which account for both the demands and, in some cases, the response by the state.

Secondly, in the cases on smoking and on water quality, the main tensions concern the relationships between government and industry. In purely liberal terms, such cases cause problems for the state because the latter is committed to protecting both the individual and the industry when the needs or demands of the two come into conflict.   However, the idea of democracy demands that if industry causes preventable harms to individuals,   then individuals have the right, under some circumstances at least, to expect the state to act in their favour. These points can help us to explain why the state acts, or does not act, in a certain way in cases such as these.

Finally, electoral short-termism was seen as important to the formulation and implementation of rational preventive policies in some of the case studies (water, breast screening, smoking and seat belts).   Here, we can see a tension between negative libertarian state approaches and the democratic demands that these things be acted upon by the state. The fact that such issues remain on the political agenda, despite the powerful libertarian forces that would see them slip off that agenda, can be seen as an illustration of the explanatory value of the ways in which a clear view of democracy can be seen to temper certain aspects of liberal ideology.

A proper and careful understanding of democracy would reveal, or so we maintain, that certain crucial provisions demand long term commitments by the very logic of democracy. This derives from the logically self-binding nature of democracy. These provisions must include, to repeat, a fundamental and egalitarian concern with the basic physical mobility of citizens. Electoral considerations, therefore, can never *rightly* get in the way of justified and effective provisions. Thus, a democratic government ought to do what it can to ensure clean water supplies equally to all its citizens regardless or short term electoral concerns. It should look likewise to the health of its citizens with regard to the use of addictive and dangerous drugs. It should also put into effect the best known means of detecting breast cancer - which must also mean forebearance where no demonstrably effective policy is yet known.

Footnotes

1) The authors would like to thank Michael Bury for his comments on an earlier draft of this chapter.

2) The terms 'liberty' and 'freedom' are used inter-changeably in this chapter.

3) See Poggi (1991) on the nature of the limited state prior to the twentieth century.

4) The policy stance of the British government's 1991 Green Paper, *The Health of the Nation*, can be explained more clearly in negative libertarian than positive libertarian terms. The need for the government to act in various ways is acknowledged. The type and extent of action, however, lays stress upon informed individuals taking responsibility for themselves. The Secretary of State's foreword notes that 'there is considerable emphasis in this document on the need for people to change their behaviour ...'. *The Observer* commented that the document relies 'almost exclusively on education and exhortation to reach the goals' (see Williams, Calnan and Cant, 1991, p. 27).

Bibliography/references

Beetham, D. (1992), 'Liberal Democracy and the Limits of Democratization', *Political Studies*, vol. XL, special issue.

Berlin, I. (1969), *Four Essays on Liberty*, Oxford University Press, Oxford.

Dahl, R.A. (1985), *A Preface to Economic Democracy*, Polity Press, Cambridge.

Elster, J. (1988), 'Introduction', in, Elster, J. and Slagstad, R. (eds), *Constitutionalism and Democracy*, Cambridge University Press, Cambridge.

Goodin, R.E. (1988), *Reasons for Welfare*, Princeton University Press, Princeton, N.J.

Held, D. (1987), *Models of Democracy*, Polity Press, Cambridge.

Lively, J. (1975), *Democracy*, Basil Blackwell, Oxford.

May, J.D. (1978), 'Defining Democracy', *Political Studies*, vol. XXVI, no. 1.

Nozick, R. (1974), *Anarchy, State and Utopia*, Basil Blackwell, Oxford.

Parekh, B. (1992), 'The Cultural Particularity of Liberal Democracy', *Political Studies*, vol. XL, special issue.

Plant, R. (1991), *Modern Political Thought*, Basil Blackwell, Oxford.

Poggi, G. (1990), *The State*, Polity Press, Cambridge.

Rawls, J. (1971), *A Theory of Justice*, Oxford University Press, Oxford.

Salecl, R. (1991), 'Democracy and Violence', *New Formations*, no. 14, Summer.

Williams, G. (1991), *Political Theory in Retrospect*, Edward Elgar, Cheltenham.
Williams, S., Calnan, M. and Cant, S. (1991), 'Health Promotion and Disease Prevention in the 1990s', *Medical Sociology News*, vol. 16, no. 3.

11   Conclusion

Mike Mills

In the previous chapter Mills and Saward picked up on a dominant theme of many of the case studies - that of ideology. Liberal democracy, it was argued, displays certain tensions when we come to consider what the proper preventive role of the state should in terms of providing services, relying on individual responsibility or acting on behalf of citizens. To a greater or lesser extent all of the cases presented here cannot be fully explained without some reference to the broader ideological framework provided by liberal democracy and, in particular, its liberal component. This framework goes a long way towards explaining which groups are seen as most deserving of state attention and which types of strategy will be preferred by the state.

But it was made clear in that chapter and in the *Introduction* that when we disaggregate prevention into its various types, other forces come into play which also help us to explain policy. While the individual and systemic approaches were particularly susceptible to ideological constraints (for example, AIDS, seat belts, smoking, water purity) they were also affected by the institutional arrangements which have been developed to decide and deliver policies (ad hoc structures, government-industry relations). Similarly, the community approach (childbirth, primary care and the development of AIDS policies) also demonstrated that institutional and professional cleavages were explanatorily important as well.

This chapter begins by considering the different levels of analysis at which we find explanations for preventive health policies and attempts to characterise the major forces which appear to shape policy. It then moves from a consideration of network theory - which provides a useful typology of political relationships - to return to ideology. I argue that should we wish to bolster the profile of prevention, we should create more open and democratic political opportunity structures.

The dominant themes of prevention

Prevention, it seems, is affected both by macro and meso-level variables. While ideology is perhaps a dominant macro theme, it is by no means the only one. Ward's chapter on water purity and Hann's on breast cancer screening touched on the cultural context within which preventive decisions are made. Even though the empirical evidence correlating risks to morbidity or mortality may be weak, cultural norms may swing decisions in favour of political action despite negligible health gains. These cases appear to suggest that cultural norms are important in our choice of preventive policies to the extent that prevention is more likely if the consequences of inaction are perceived to touch upon entrenched social fears, particularly those associated with issues of symbolic importance (water) or vulnerability (cancers). In cases such as these we may be able to explain, for example, apparent inconsistencies in the political prominence given to low level or unmanageable risks through their cultural significance. Culture, though important to the political context in which decisions are made, has to be used cautiously in political explanation. Elans and Simeon, for example, argue that cultural variables should be used sparingly and only once we have established that other factors, institutions and structural variables for example, cannot in themselves provide adequate explanations (Elans and Simeon, 1979). This is not to dismiss culture, but rather to suggest that the policy dynamic may lay elsewhere.

It was clear from the cases of smoking, water purity, and the EC that broader economic considerations (the effects of prevention on producer and capital interests) do constrain the actions of the state. However, we have to be careful in the conclusions that we draw as far as the affect of economic constraints are concerned. On one level it is clear that governments do consider the effects of policies on wider economic issues - Bomberg and Peterson, for example, showed how European countries were acutely aware of the effects that auto-emission regulations would have on their domestic auto-manufacturing industries. Ward gave us a very good example of how the Thatcher government was constrained in its water privatisation policy by the knowledge that the share floatation would fail if investment in the industry, and promises of price increases above the rate of inflation, were not forthcoming. Having said this, there is a difference between the broad structural constraints experienced by governments from economic\capital interests and the activities of producer interests on the other. The former is a macro-level constraint which all British (and other) governments face. By definition a structural is not something which need be articulated, but rather, is simply an inherent constraint upon policy makers. The latter concerns the specific actions of producers on particular issues. Producers, while invariabley aware of their structural economic importance, nevertheless transform that structural economic position into representation in decision making centres - of course, governments are often instrumental in achieving such incorporation. In short, one of the great political benefits enjoyed by producer and capital interests is that they enjoy not only a structural advantage as far as their position in the domestic economy goes but, as a consequence of this, their position within the decision making process is also augmented. At both levels the considerations of producers and governments are roughly the same, although precisely how these considerations manifest themselves in response to preventive issues is a much messier business.

The evidence of the case studies leads us to suppose that producer interests are sensitive to the association of their product with adverse health consequences and it is this which acts as the focus for their political actions. This much, perhaps, is obvious but it is evident that we need to know a little more about the calculations of producers before such a supposition becomes of much use.

On one level it is apparent that there is a coincidence of interest between producers and consumers of, say, food. Consumers want good, wholesome food, and producers want to avoid consumers suffering as a consequence of eating their products. This does not, however, help us to explain those instances when producers defend their products (as the dairy industry have done) when the evidence appears to suggest that consumers will suffer from their consumption.

It is more accurate to argue, though, that producers have an interest in avoiding adverse health consequences being *attributed* to their products - this is a strategy which has been employed in the past by the tobacco and food industries. The tendency amongst producer interests is to emphasise that individuals choose whether to, for example, drink alcohol and which foods to eat and it is only the manner (or extent) to which we do this which causes us problems - hence the argument that diseases of the late 20th century are diseases of affluence. In short, there is nothing inherently wrong with the products offered for sale, only the way they are consumed. In addition, of course, producers are able to exploit the regular divisions of opinion between 'experts' on what these adverse health consequences are supposed to be or, more importantly, what their causes are. It is, for example, known that saturated fat is a risk factor for heart disease, but very difficult to demonstrate that saturated fat, as opposed to one of the other risk factors, does a person harm.

It is the question of attribution, rather than wholesale product defence, which explains why producers will exploit equivocal empirical evidence relating their products to adverse health consequences in consumers. Equally, attribution sensitises us to the fact that prevention cannot be based upon the assumption that a cast iron coincidence of interests between consumers and producers exists - this does not work when 1) producers are in a monopoly position (e.g. water); 2) consumers are addicted to products (e.g. tobacco); or 3) when it is producers who decide whether a risk is associated with their product (e.g. food). If we are looking for generalisation which will hold across preventive issues, then attribution is a much better description of producer calculations than any suggestion that producers are either consumer-friendly full-stop, or simply unscrupulous.

Secondly, even if we know that preventive health policies will, if adopted, adversely affect economic interests, this is unlikely to tell us what the political response of industry will be. Take, for example, the cases of seat belts and the regulation of tobacco products. Despite the fact that requiring the fitting of seat belts would increase the costs of cars, there is little if any evidence that motor manufacturers or retailers seemed to worry about this. On the other hand, the tobacco industry, also faced with having to raise its prices (admittedly to a greater extent), fights tooth and nail. In the case of seat belts, producer interests were queuing up to endorse their adoption because many industries would benefit from fewer accidents on the road (not least the brewers). But with tobacco there is nothing of any merit that can be done to improve the product and the only realistic option open to producers is a damage limitation strategy. Again we return to the notion that it is in the calculations of producers that they must minimise the adverse health consequences attributed to their products - alcohol gets a bad press when associated with deaths or injuries on the roads so do the manufacturers of cars.

Thirdly, the simple formula which argues that producers want to protect their profits is a little too simple. If, for example, government had tried to introduce seat belts only into the 'riskiest' cars (which tend to be small cars) then there would not have been the consensus amongst producers that there was. The effects would have been the same if legislation was passed to fit seat belts into Fords but not into Vauxhalls. In short, while producers will always be reluctant to incur an absolute increase in their costs, they are much more concerned that their position in relation to their competitors is not disadvantaged. By implication prevention, to the extent that it does require product regulation to be changed, stands a much greater chance of being accepted by producers if its commercial disadvantages are spread fairly between competitors. Given that these competitors are not only domestic but also members of the international economy, then the need for regulation at the international level would seem evident if this problem is to be overcome. The deliberations surrounding the introduction of a carbon tax in Britain is a very good illustration of this. But the difficulties are obvious. It is hardly possible to treat the competitors of the butter manufacturing industry fairly if we withdraw EC sudsidies on butter - it is clear that margarine manufacturers will benefit. Similarly, increasing the excise on drinks with a high alcohol content cannot be done fairly as far as the manufacturers of those drinks are concerned.

The point is that the calculations of economic interests are complex - sometimes it is in their interests to fight preventive policies, at other times it is better to embrace them. In general, producers will fight regulation when they perceive that their competitive position and/or the integrity of their products, cannot survive the adoption of preventive policies - Bomberg and Peterson's case study of automobile manufacturers and the EC is a very good case in point.

But we also have to accept that these constraints are mediated politically, in other words, that it is often the state, as much as economic interests themselves, which perceives a constraint to exist. For example, it would be unwise to suggest that the government were any less aware of the problems associated with the privatisation of the water industry, than the prospective buyers were.

We are left in the position, therefore, of arguing that the broader economic framework within which preventive policies are made and adopted is crucially affected by two things - the competitive nature of the economic system itself (which constrains the actions of both the state and producer/capital interests) and the trade-offs that the state must make between economic and, in our case, health interests. This applies both at the level of a broad structural constraint acting on policy makers, and at the (meso) level where producers argue their own case. Each of these are largely concerned with the individual and systemic aspects of prevention because it is these strategies which are more likely to affect our behaviour as consumers and, hence, also affect the market place. Because the community approach tends to work within a series of fairly autonomous systems - and crucially, has little market impact - the factors which affect it are different, as we saw in the *Introduction*.

This makes it very difficult to predict precisely how economic interests in general will respond to preventive policies and what effect they will have on them. What we can say with some authority is that these interests will be reluctant to attribute health problems to their products if they can avoid doing so and they will resist regulation which leaves them at a competitive disadvantage. This does not mean, however, that they will not incur costs if they perceive it is in the interests to do so. The dynamic which explains the actions of both the state and producers as far as economic constraints are concerned, pivots around the twin notions of competitiveness and the absolute ability of industry to incur increased costs.

Fragmentation and network theory

We are getting closer to understanding the political nature of preventive health policies because we can see that the interaction of macro-level variables is complex and difficult to predict. But it was argued earlier that at the meso-level any policy inconsistencies are magnified, not least because of the fragmentary nature of preventive policy making.

Throughout the case studies we have seen that institutional structures (smoking, primary care, AIDS), professional cleavages (AIDS, primary care, childbirth), divisions in departmental responsibilities (smoking) and policy territoriality (EC) can significantly affect preventive policies. These are, of course, factors in all policy making but are particularly important to preventive policies because prevention touches upon so many areas of public policy which do not have health as their primary focus.

Policy fragmentation, therefore, is a political problem. We know that the ethos of prevention is not applied with any consistency across policy areas and given the diversity of preventive policies this may be unsurprising. Having said this, it would be wrong to think that we can make no sense of the fragmentary nature of policy making. We can, at the very least, apply labels to the types of policy making relationships that do exist, and in doing so, gain some insights into, and explanations of, our case studies.

In recent years a great deal of work has been done on disaggregating the different types of political relationships which can affect policy. For our purposes, the work done in network theory appears to provide a very good description of many of the cases presented here.

Network theory tells us that we should not view policy making as a uniform, monolithic exercise, in the same way that I have indicated that there is no single preventive strategy. The work of people such as Rhodes (1986, 1988), Wilks and Wright (1987), Grant et al.(1988), and Laffin (1986) emphasises the fact that policy making varies along many different lines and that we should expect different parts of the state, and perhaps even different parts of the same government department, to operate in a unique way.

By and large what authors agree most upon is the need to disaggregate and to understand the peculiarities of policy making in any given setting, but beyond this, there is much less agreement. Both conceptually and methodologically there is disagreement on how far to disaggregate and what the precise meanings of concepts are. For this reason I have chosen to focus largely upon the work of Rhodes, primarily because his model does offer the opportunity to incorporate many of the factors which appear important to preventive policies.

Rhodes argues that there are discernible patterns of political relationships which operate at the sub-sectoral level and which can form a typology that covers most policy making eventualities. The typology looks like this:

Policy communities - are generally tightly knit networks of actors who have a very focused interest in an aspect of policy. This small group or clique controls policy and will only allow new members into the group if they can be fairly sure they will not rock the boat. In other words, the entry qualifications are quite strict, the membership is stable, there is a strong degree of value consensus and power is concentrated, although it is the representatives of government who should have the most power. The relationship between the National Farmers Union (NFU) and the Ministry of Agriculture Fisheries and Food (MAFF) is a classic example of a policy community.

Professionalised networks - are dominated by one particular type of interest, professionals. Again, if decisions are being made largely by professionals, as was the case with doctors in the NHS for example, then we have strict entry qualifications to this group, we assume a certain level of cohesion within the network because of the shared training and work experiences of doctors, and we also expect this to be a reasonably exclusive type of network. We would not necessarily expect to find the network located within a particular government department, it is much more likely that a professionalised network, and its influence, would be spread throughout an organisation.

Producer networks - are similar to professionalised networks in that they are patterns of political relationships but which are dominated by producer interests - Read gave us the example of the tobacco industry. Here, it is the common interests that producers have in a policy which motivates them to 'network' either formally or informally in order to influence policy. Grant et al. (1988), provide some interesting examples of this for government-chemical industry relations in Britain and Germany. Producer networks simply recognise the fact that it is possible to discern producers working together or with government to create a pattern of relationships, understandings and agreed norms which they then use of affect public policy.

By and large it is these three types of network that we are interested in, although there are two others identified by Rhodes which deserve a mention. The first is *territorial communities*, where the network of interests is restricted and focuses on territorial interests; and the second is *issues networks* where actors tend to move in and out of the policy arena quite frequently, where there is very little value consensus amongst participants and hence less overtly political control over policy.

It is not difficult to see at a glance that many of our case studies do fit this typology quite well. Lane's chapter on homebirths, for example, emphasises the fact that the procedures for giving birth have been professionally captured and it is the position of health professionals within the health care system which allows them to continue to determine policy on homebirths. Consequently, it is useful to describe the pattern of relationships which doctors have over the nature and location of giving birth, as a professionalised network. Hann's chapter on breast cancer screening also demonstrates the ability of professionals to form networks of expertise and, as a consequence, perhaps narrow the range of advice or opinions to government. Here, the network is formed around certain medical issues and involves professional elites - nevertheless, a professionalised network still exists. Street's chapter on AIDS tells a very similar story in which there clearly were networks of professional interests involved in the development of policies. Street also argued that AIDS policy was effectively captured by those with clinical skills, while members of the Health Education Advisory Group and the Terrence Higgins Trust were marginalised even though their own expertise might be expected to be central to policy. Again, the concept of a professionalised network controlling access to decision making centres would seem appropriate.

Policy communities occur both in Read's chapter on smoking and Bomberg and Peterson's chapter on the EC. Read explicitly argued that the tobacco lobby had formed a policy community within the DoH which was dedicated to the protection of the industry itself. What is perhaps most interesting about Read's case is how it demonstrates the level of isolation that policy communities can experience from the broader social value base. There are a number of eminent professional and charity groups chipping away at this particular government-industry relationship, and yet the industry has managed to embed itself very deeply (and very deliberately) into the very structure of the state.

Bomberg and Peterson also allude to policy communities within the EC, where the tendency towards territoriality provides a good microcosm of the fragmentary nature of policy making in many large political organisations. They specifically argued that this tendency does hinder a more general policy on prevention because of the way these policy communities insulate themselves from outside interference. It is not difficult to see that this could have an effect on the way policy is made because policy communities evolve precisely because policy is perceived to need tight control and because there are very specific lines along which it should run.

When we look at the examples of AIDS and seat belts we see that the idea of an issue network has some plausibility. The passage of legislation in Parliament, particularly on a free vote, does indicate that procedurally and institutionally policy was a free-for-all in which the usual political constraints exerted by government were, in some instances at least, diluted. Similarly, it is not unreasonable to suppose that, when AIDS first became a political issue, policy was subject to a very broad range of interests before settling down into a more formal and controlled pattern of political control.

Thus far it is possible to see the utility of using a typology such as this particularly when we explore its implications for the nature of preventive policies themselves. Network theory suggests that each network will have its own 'rules of the game' which political participants will need to know and abide by; it suggests that while there may be acknowledged ideologically consistencies across policy areas there is likely to be a co-existing value consensus within each network which would make each of them unique and which would filter any broader structural or ideological constraints.

Preventive health policies vary, then, in a number of key respects. On the basis of network theory we would expect that preventive policies would find it particularly difficult to break into policy areas which are dominated by a policy community unless the preventive aspects of policy are already part of the value consensus.

Similarly, while we would expect that the value consensus within some professionalised networks would be geared to health, we cannot say that even within the NHS prevention is central to the professional ethos. Allsop and Freeman argued that the health care system is not imbued with a preventive orientation, and highlighted the way in which institutional changes over the past twenty years had done little to change this. The strength of health professionals has to a great extent resided in their ability to create and manage a network based upon a predominantly bio-medical model of health. Indeed, many of the more overtly political aspects of the recent reforms can be seen as an attempt by the state to reduce the scope of this network and confine it to a stricter definition of clinical (as opposed to managerial) autonomy. Lane's chapter on childbirth tells much the same story as far as the ability of professionals to control policy goes.

Furthermore, it was argued in the *Introduction* that professionalisation, and the consequent professional networks, has a strong institutional aspect - that is, these networks operate within institutions which accommodate the level of control and autonomy necessary for professionalism to exist. On this basis, it is not unreasonable to argue that if political relationships are enduring, we are likely to see them express themselves in some kind of monument or testimony to the balance of political forces at the time. In the case of the tobacco industry we have codes of practice which define and legitimise the activities of the industry; in the case of health professionals we have had reforms of the health care system which institutionally advantage and promote one type of health care strategy over and above others.

In short, network theory does help us to understand; 1) that preventive policies are fragmented (something which is perhaps obvious anyway); 2) that networks are built around political relationships predicated upon certain assumptions about the nature of the participants (they won't rock the boat); 3) that networks have no real incentive to change themselves and we should expect the source of policy change to come from the outside; 4) that they have a tendency to anchor themselves in place by producing policies, structures or procedures which express their own political, professional, producer or territorial interests; 5) that even if we can identify macro-level imperatives which affect preventive policies, these will always be filtered through values, institutions and political resources which actually deal with the elimination, detection, prediction or management of societal risks.

The work of Wilks and Wright (1987) also suggests that networks can account for the effects of agency (individuals) on policy. In the cases of public health (Allsop and Freeman, chapter 2) and AIDS (Street, chapter 5) we saw that although we can identify broad macro and meso-level constraints on, and facilities for, policy, we cannot give a full explanation of these cases without reference to the actions of individuals. In other words, micro-level analysis is also important.

In both of these cases it was the Chief Medical Officer (CMO), Sir Donald Acheson, who seemed to make a material difference to the development of policies. This is important because meso-level analysis would suggest that it is the office of CMO which is important - because it provides certain resources to the incumbent - not the person who holds the office. Yet we have found that the ability of individuals to influence policies is not confined to the power (resources) provided by the office. It is unlikely that policies on AIDS and public health would have developed in the way they did and at the time they did with a different CMO. Having said this, of course, the public health initiative did succumb to the fragmentation associated with departmental territorial interests, and AIDS policy was eventually captured by the clinicians - both of these outcomes are highly predictable when using a meso and/or macro framework.

*   *   *   *   *

The suggestion is that the cases presented here need to be explained on two different levels. Firstly, we cannot avoid the conclusions drawn in the previous chapter that the dominant liberal democratic ideology has a profound effect on preventive health policies. Similarly, our cases suggest that the structural effects of economic constraints are also profound, certainly as far as the individual and systemic approaches to prevention are concerned. However, other countries are liberal democracies and have economies as well, but respond differently to the same political imperatives. Consequently, we have to look to the types of institutional arrangements that Britain displays, its policy 'style', our culture and the participatory opportunities which are afforded to groups, to explain away the differences between ourselves and others. Here we find that these broader macro-level imperatives are filtered through cleavages which are endemic to preventive policies, but which seem to be exacerbated by the autonomy afforded to professionals at all political levels, the informal but highly restrictive nature of our decision making process (which is characterised well by network theory) and the limited opportunities afforded to 'outsider' groups to scrutinise or participate in decision making.

In the *Introduction* I posed three questions, the answers to which appeared to provide some justification for considering prevention, health and British politics. These questions were: is it possible to generalise about the nature of prevention or preventive policies; do concepts which are normally associated with prevention (risk and vulnerability for example) help us to explain across policy areas; what are the political constraints and opportunities which an essentially preventive health care strategy faces; and do certain types of prevention have greater political mileage than others?

We are now in a position to give answers to these questions, albeit tentative at times. Risk and vulnerability are important to the extent that the latter is defined through cultural and ideological factors which tend to promote perceptions of some groups (women and children for example) as more deserving and more vulnerable than others. In turn this goes some way to explaining the patriarchal nature of policies related to homebirths. Risk, as Douglas and Wildavsky argued, is socially constructed, but just as importantly, it is also politically mediated and hence is very bad at explaining preventive health policies. The exception to this comes when the risks are perceived to be acute, as was the case with breast cancer screening, for example, and the food scares of the late 1980s. Of course, these perceptions are themselves often politically mediated and socially constructed. We can generalise about the nature and policies of prevention to the extent that we can identify imperatives which affect those policies, but these vary in their effects according to the approach to prevention which is adopted, the political interests which are involved and the institutional structures which are in place. Certain approaches to prevention do appear to be more popular with governments than others - the individual approach serves many purposes besides that of providing information or education and in the past has been used as a substitute for the more expensive community approach and the more politically sensitive systemic approach. In short, prevention reflects very well the dominant political, ideological, economic and cultural aspects of our political system - the shortcomings of one, are the shortcomings of the other.

Prevention and democracy revisited

It was never the intention of this book to actively prescribe preventive health policies as inherently preferable to more curative approaches. Having said this, it is evident that where prevention can be of some benefit we are entitled, if not obliged, to assess the reasons why it struggles for acceptance amongst policy makers. At the very least we have set ourselves the task of looking for generalisations and explanations of what we have found in the case studies.

It is not unreasonable, therefore, to take this a stage further and to explore, or re-explore, some of the fundamental tenets of policy to unravel where the particular obstacles and opportunities fall. It is here that the theoretical arguments given in this chapter do more than simply allow us to describe the case studies in a different way.

In the previous chapter, Mills and Saward, argued that much of the prevention with which our case studies have been concerned can be explained in terms of the values, responsibilities and structures inherent in liberal democracy. I want to return to these types of arguments in this final section.

The literature on prevention, or preventive policy areas, consistently produces evidence that certain features of our political and economic system constrain or actively inhibit preventive health policies - Allsop and Freeman gave us a thorough account of these factors, as have the *Introduction* and *Conclusion*. Liberal democracy, however, is much more concerned with principles, rather than the practice of policy, but is influential nevertheless.

It seems to me that this ideology, or the imbalance between its (none too compatible) parts is at the core of preventions problem in Britain. Chapter 10 alerted us to the fact that while liberalism suggests that protection of freedoms or liberties formed a central consideration of policy makers, it was the democratic values of our political organisation and the more positive libertarian trend in liberal thinking which prompted the state to take on more than minimal responsibilities for our well being. Reducing this to a couple of key features, this entails; the state ascribing rights greater than those necessary for the minimalist 'freedom from' state coercion, in other words some form of social rights; the state creating the conditions (human) under which citizens can perform their democratic responsibilities (for example, basic education and mobility); the state accepting that the process of democracy entails some notion of responsiveness to the demands of citizens; the opportunity to articulate demands and opportunities to participate politically.

The emphasis which was placed upon ideology as an explanatory variable has been an emphasis of its liberal aspect - in other words, it is the preponderance of liberal values which explains much preventive health policy. Conversely, then, I would suggest that should we wish to resolve this problem (if, of course, it is perceived to be a problem) then it is to the democratic element of our ideology that we must turn.

While such things as fragmentation, professional cleavages, the use of experts, the _pulation of scientific evidence and government-industry relations are all important in explaining preventive health policies, we are still left with the problem of what we do in response to them. My suggestion is that we do not argue for the reversal of these trends in particular, but rather, for the democratisation of the system within which these policies are formulated and implemented.

Why is democracy the problem? Let me return for a second to the description of networks given in the previous section. Networks were only used as a shorthand method of describing the sorts of political relationships which appear to affect preventive health policies, whether the strategies used are individual, community or systemic. What was important about these descriptions, as far as prevention was concerned, was the exclusive and restricted nature of their membership and the control they had over policy. Whether we were dealing with professionals in the NHS, producer interests around the DoH or another government department, or policy communities in the EC, each demonstrated what we might call a democratic deficit. In other words, it is the absence of public scrutiny, limited public or group access, little public accountability and a lack of political responsiveness by government which are absent in the policy making procedure.

Our case studies suggest that many of the barriers to prevention rely upon the persistence of ideological, economic and institutional predispositions which would find it hard to 'live with' an opening up of the decision making process. The NHS, for example, has always been a remarkably undemocratic institution with very little in the way of scrutiny and accountability to either central government or its clients. The current reforms emphasise that accountability is to be primarily economic in nature but the deficit which has orientated the system away from prevention and which, for example, has institutionalised births within hospitals, is much more a political deficit - hence Lane's argument for participation rather than professionalisation. A similar story of 'capture' is told in policies on AIDS. While we can explain policies with a combination of party ideology and professional networking, it was the paucity of genuine participatory opportunities which excluded interests such as the Terrence Higgins Trust and the Health Education Advisory Group from policy centres. Tobacco industry relations with government, the investment in the water industry before privatisation and the network of professionals which built up around the issue of breast cancer screening all suggest that one or more of the key elements of democracy were missing from the decision making process.

Much the same type of argument can be used when we turn to the evidence upon which political decisions are made. We know that empirical evidence goes through many incarnations before it reaches the stage of policy (if it reaches that stage). We also know that it is argued over, suppressed, used for politically expedient purposes (e.g. just before a general election) and ignored. Consequently the correlation between levels of risk and policy is very low indeed. It is not, I think, stretching a point too far to suggest that a more open, participatory and informative polity might overcome some of these problems. This is not to say that our policies on food or alcohol, for example, would be very different, but it would mean that the political (preventive) choices which were being made became more explicit. Preventive policies, like all other policies, are a question of political choice. Again, this would not necessarily promote prevention per se, but would challenge many of the reasons why we fail to adopt preventive health policies.

Furthermore, we can pick up on a point made by Allsop and Freeman whic have important democratic consequences - their comparison between the British on prevention and the records of north American and Scandinavian countries. These unfavourable comparisons can be drawn because the political opportunity structures in Britain are so good at syphoning off dissent without conceding a great deal at the level of policy. In other words, our system of government is not open enough to allow the types of social democratic participation that exist in Scandinavia, nor liberal enough to encourage active citizenship, as in north America. Indeed, a large part of Cunningham's explanation for development of these policies rested upon just these sorts of ideas.

The apparent inconsistencies that we have found in the political responses to societal risks are as much inconsistencies in our democratic framework, as they are a reflection of anything inherent in the risks themselves. The assumptions of democracy, therefore, do not require us to adopt preventive health policies simply because they are 'preventive', but they challenge us to consider whether we are satisfied with the explanations for those policies.

Bibliography\references

Douglas, M. and Wildavsky, A. (1982), *Risk and Culture*, University of California Press, Berkeley.

Elkins, D. and Simeon, R. (1979), 'A cause in search of its effect, or what does political culture explain?', *Comparative Politics*, vol. 11, pp. 127-45.

Laffin, M. (1986), *Professionalism and Power*, Gower, Aldershot.

Grant, W. et al. (1988), *Government and the Chemical Industry*, Oxford University Press, London.

Rhodes, R.A.W., (1986), *The National World of Local Government*, Allen and Unwin, London.

Rhodes, R A W (1988), *Beyond Westminster and Whitehall*, Unwin Hyman, London

Wilks, S. and Wright, M. (eds) (1987), *Comparative Government-Industry Relations*, Clarendon Press, Oxford.

Index

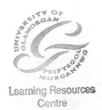